TAPPING THE FOUNTAIN OF YOUTH

PROFILES OF WOMEN RUNNERS OVER 50

CAROL HANSEN MONTGOMERY

2012

DEDICATION

This book is dedicated to my son, David Fenichel,
who ran the Boston Marathon by my side,
and
Herbert Townsend, my partner,
who keeps me running.

CONTENTS

Acknowledgements.................................... vii

Foreword ix

Chapter 1: Introduction 1

Chapter 2: Ages 50–54 7
Carole O. Donohue.............................7
Lillian Feliciano 14
Abby Raven 19
Susan Reich.. 25

Chapter 3: Ages 55–59 31
Carol Ardell 31
Nancy L. Smith 38
Dori Iten... 44
Carolyn R. Bujak...................................50

Chapter 4: Ages 60–64 57
Suzanne Gibson................................... 57
Diane McManus................................... 64
Mary Kessler 71
Joy Hampton 78

Chapter 5: Ages 65–69 83
Sue Baker..83
Millie Hamilton....................................90
Freddi Carlip 97
Carole Lelli 103

Chapter 6: Ages 70–74 111
Sue Levy..111
Sandra Folzer 115
Gloria Jenkins...................................... 120
Rita Alles.. 125

Chapter 7: Ages 75–79 .... **131**
    Mary Harada 131
    Carol Montgomery 136
    Zandra Moeburg-Price 143
    Katherine Beiers 149

Chapter 8: Ages 80 Plus **155**
    Lois Ann Gilmore 155
    Madonna Buder 160
    Betty Lundquist 167
    Jackie Yost 172

Glossary **179**

ACKNOWLEDGEMENTS

Foremost, I would like to acknowledge the outstanding work of Mike MacKay in photographing many of the women in this book and editing photos of the others to their maximum potential. Key to this effort was the assistance of Mike's triathlete wife, Marian, who assisted with the photo shoots and gave up a lot of time with her husband during their "winter holiday" in Florida. This book is vastly improved because of their involvement. See Mike's work at www.mikemackay.ca.

I want to express enormous gratitude to Kathrine Switzer for writing the Foreword. Her encouragement and involvement were invaluable. Kathrine's friend, Jenny Hadfield, provided help at a critical time.

I also want to thank Adrienne Moch, who assisted with the writing, and Ben Asher for his very able copy editing. Both are superb professionals.

Less direct, but key, was the training of my coach, Mike Patterson, without whom I would never have developed as a runner to the place where I could write this book.

Finally, all of the amazing women profiled here gave willingly of their valuable time and energy. None held back in telling their stories.

I've been running for 53 years. I just turned 65, and I swear to you, some days I still feel like that 12-year-old-girl who is learning how to run and is thrilled with the discovery of herself. Because every day, running is *still* a discovery!

Yet, how will I be running in five years? Ten years? Will I be running at all in ten years?

Let's put it this way: I'm counting on it. Already there have been plenty of changes in my running, and there are others ahead for me, but what are they? How much speed will I lose? Can I retain my great endurance? Or, will I have to stop because of injuries or simply because I'm just "too old"? (Perish the thought!)

These are questions that all dedicated runners ask themselves at some time, most often while out for an easy jog, and certainly if the exercise begins to take more effort or time. Lucky for us, the questions can be addressed by looking to older runners as role models.

Until very recently, we runners—women especially—have had few role models over the age of 50. During the running boom of the 1970s, it was rare to find women runners even in their 40s. Now in most small local races it is unusual to find women over 60.

Tapping the Fountain of Youth: Profiles of Women Runners Over 50 is important because it fills this information void. The few articles in mainstream running publications about older women nearly always focus on a single exceptionally accomplished woman. Certainly they inspire us! But even for me, with a lifetime of experience, they can be hard to relate to. The stories in this book are told by Carol Hansen Montgomery, a 70-something sprite who has been part of the running movement for 35 years. Carol feels it, and understand it, and brings us these delightful, inspiring, and totally relatable stories of women with a range of abilities and experiences. Only one started running shortly after college. Several started running in their 50s and—more amazingly—in their 60s. The message: It really is never too late.

These are the very women who inspired me to question my own ability when I turned 60. Although a lifetime daily runner, I'd stopped marathoning three decades (yes, 30 years!) before to concentrate on my career and books. Then I began meeting more and more women who were just beginning to run in their 60s—even 70s—and they propelled me back into testing myself again at the marathon distance. Yes! I did it! Proving another message: It's never too late to get it back.

This book is important also because it is written for a large and rapidly growing audience. Female runners outnumbered men in all U.S. road races in 2010 up to the marathon distance, and in the 18–39 age group in the 2011 Boston Marathon. There were seven million female road racers in 2010, up from one million in 2000. All of these women should read this book at some time in their running lives, because guess what? Ready or not, we're going to get older. So—be ready. And enjoy the ride as well as the destination.

Be fearless. Be free.

Kathrine Switzer
Author, *Marathon Woman*
First woman to officially enter and run the Boston Marathon

CHAPTER 1: INTRODUCTION

In 2010, Gladys Burrill, 92, finished the Honolulu Marathon, setting a Guinness World Record for the oldest woman to complete the distance. In the same year, Mary Harada, 75, ran a 7:55 mile to set the world mark for women 75–79; and Susan Reich, 52, was the female winner of the Ocean City Half Marathon and fifth overall in a field of 325. In 2012, Joy Hampton, 65, completed her 25th consecutive Boston Marathon, placing in the top 10 in her age group every year since turning 60 and finishing second three times..

Are these ladies exceptional? They most certainly are, since the senior women who excel as runners today didn't have the opportunities girls now have. Their high-school and college years preceded the passage of Title IX in 1972, which increased opportunities for women to participate in scholastic and college sports. Most began to run in their 30s and 40s and later. Or, if they were athletes at a younger age, they often interrupted their sports activities to raise families before returning to competition.

This book features interviews with 28 women in their 50s and beyond who run and compete in races. These women range from international-class competitive athletes to recreational runners. While each has a unique, inspiring story, they're also collectively, in a sense, "everywoman." They're single, married, working, retired—from different races and ethnicities. Some have children, grandchildren, or even great-grandchildren. They're survivors who may have experienced loss, illness, or personal crises...and find in their running a new strength to cope with these trials.

Why They Run

What have these women found as runners that keeps them going? What can readers learn from their longevity in competition? Perhaps the key lesson is that many limits people set are artificial and that with proper self-care, we not only can extend our lives, but enhance our vitality. While men have often grown up being encouraged to be athletic, most of the women featured here discovered their athletic potential later in life—several as late as age 60. Earlier, they may have encountered social biases against women in sports, being told that such pursuits were not "ladylike," and possibly even damaging. Thus, they had to face and overcome both gender and age barriers—yet this didn't stop them.

The examples they set can offer an object lesson to other women who face similar obstacles.

They came to running for many reasons: to enjoy the health and fitness benefits of exercise, to relieve stress, to keep off weight. And they stayed. Running can be seductive that way. Walk into any running store, and you'll find race entry forms and running-club announcements. Buy a pair of shoes, and you've bought into a culture. Enter one race, and you'll find opportunities to enter more. A new world opens up, one that someone past 50 with children in high school or college—or on her own—has more time to enjoy. Surprisingly to most women interviewed, new friendships form based on running. Some have even found husbands and life partners in the running community.

Fortunately, these friendships aren't dependent on speed. Most running clubs are open to runners regardless of ability, with faster members waiting at races and cheering on those finishing later. Racing offers the chance to experience crowd support once reserved for the elite. And while slowing down may be part of the aging process, age-group and age-graded competition allow runners to compete on a level playing field with their peers.

Indeed, a major factor bringing older runners into races is age-group competition. While road racing is hardly new—the Boston Marathon has been contested since 1897—the upsurge in popularity of running for fitness spawned more road-race choices from the 5K to the marathon. With these races came a greater interest among runners in testing themselves against not the fastest of the field, but against their peers, and so arose age-group competition.

Woman Power

As increasing numbers of women entered races, they raised awareness of women's athletic potential. Barred since the 1928 Olympics from any distance over 400 meters due to a perception that they were too delicate to handle more, women pushed the boundaries. Before Title IX made girls' teams available, women such as Doris Brown Heritage, a middle-distance standout as early as the 1960s, trained with men. Joan Benoit, while able to join girls' and women's teams, was still aware of the bias against females training. For example, while training on roads early on, she reports, "I'd walk when cars passed me. I'd pretend I was looking at the flowers."

Benoit didn't let this bias prevent her from entering and winning the female division of the 1979 Boston Marathon, a race that only opened officially to women in 1972. Roberta Gibb was the first woman to run it unofficially in 1966, and in 1967 Kathrine Switzer succeeded in entering officially by listing only her initials on the race application form. So strong was the race director's feeling that women did not belong in the race that he tried to forcibly remove her. Fortunately, he was unsuccessful.

Slowly, gender barriers fell. The 800-meter run was reopened to women in the 1960 Olympics, and the 1500, marathon, and 10K were added in 1972, 1984, and 1988, respectively. In response to the comparative lack of track opportunities for women, the Road Runners Club of America set up the Women's Distance Festival in 1979, a series of 5K races held in a variety of locations nationwide, to encourage women to run. Although women now often outnumber men in road races, the Women's Distance Festival continues to provide all-women's racing opportunities today.

The pivotal and defining event for women's running in the U.S. was Benoit's dramatic win in the 1984 women's Olympic marathon, the first time the race was offered for women. As Diane McManus describes it, "I stayed glued to the TV. As Joan Benoit widened her lead, flying through the streets of Los Angeles, I was in awe; here was a woman so focused, so fast. When she crossed the finish line as the winner, it was a victory for all women athletes—or aspiring athletes—a defining moment not only for women's sports, but for women."

With increasing opportunities for younger women came opportunities for their elders. Ruth Anderson reports that the AAU (precursor to USA Track & Field) set up a Women's and Masters Long Distance Committee in 1975, and the first World Veterans Athletics Championships (now the World Masters Athletics Championships) were contested. Since then, masters participation has grown significantly, encompassing athletes in their 50s, 60s, 70s, and older. In fact, the USA Track & Field website currently features record performances through the 100–104 age group for men and the 95–99 age group for women. Given the improvements in training and sports medicine for older athletes, it wouldn't be surprising for women to set records at age 100 and over.

Defying Age Stereotypes

This book features women who haven't allowed age to hold them back from seeking their potential as athletes. While competition in the higher age groups has increased, so has the obesity rate in the U.S. At the same time that some older women are defying the limits, others impose them as they age, dismissing the idea of strenuous exercise. They see age, weight, concern about health, or fear of injury as barriers. Although running may not be everyone's first choice of sport, the lessons that over-50 women runners can offer to other senior women are that we can embrace an active life, we have greater energy than we imagine, and turning 50 or 60 or 70 or even 80 doesn't necessarily consign us to the ranks of spectators.

While competitive success—and the pride that comes with it—is a motivating theme in all lives of the women we profile, it's only one reason to run. Dori Iten perhaps put it best: "The self-confidence carries over to other areas of my life." Several women used running to stop smoking. "Not wanting to gain weight" was mentioned almost universally. And staying slender, of course, led to good health and an appearance, some would claim, 10 years younger than their sedentary friends. (Check the photos to judge for yourself.) Abby Raven says, "A nice unexpected benefit of running is that I look younger than most women my age. My husband tells me that I don't look so good by accident. He knows how hard I work at it." Abby adds, "It's more than vanity. I'm looking for balance. I view exercise as part of a healthy life. Without it, there's something missing."

That feeling of "something missing" or "a void" is what happens to all these women when they can't exercise. Carol Lelli puts it this way: "I'm addicted to exercise and that is a good thing." What happens when these women are injured and can't run? They bike, swim, and go to the gym to use the elliptical trainer or StairMaster®, or spin. One ran in deep water without a flotation device for 10 minutes; another, in a cast that made her leg immobile, used a hula hoop.

This type of resilience, determination, and resourcefulness "runs" through these women's stories. All have suffered running injuries to some extent. And all but one—an 80-year-old who competes in tennis tournaments—have come back, often many times. Through both research and trial and error they've developed strategies to prevent future injuries: increased rest days, less running and more cross-training, strength training. Some see chiropractors, acupuncturists, or massage therapists regularly.

These women continue to challenge themselves. Several became accomplished triathletes as well as excellent runners. A few decided marathons weren't hard enough and ran ultras of 50 miles. To quote Carole Donohue: "When I turned 50, I thought what could be more appropriate than to run a 50-mile ultra?" Diane McManus describes a 5.25-mile swim race in open water: "By three miles, the water was getting choppier, and I became seasick. As the swim progressed, I felt worse. Still, I finished. My confidence soared; I could hang in through seasickness and finish something most people hadn't done. Many have run marathons. Not so many can swim that far across open water."

Perhaps nowhere does these women's determination show up more than in their efforts to run the Boston Marathon. Boston is special because of the requirement to qualify by running a certified marathon in a specified time that's determined by the runner's age and sex. Boston is the Holy Grail for marathoners and most don't find it easy to qualify or to run it. As Suzanne Gibson tells it, "I had to go to Boston. And then running became not quite so much fun. I needed to train hard. Running through the winter was tough. I had to train in the dark. It was cold and lonely. I worked all day as a nurse and then ran 10 miles many nights."

The Running Lifestyle

One of the most fun aspects of a running life is to combine it with travel. Carol Ardell says, "Traveling is one of the best aspects of this sport; we travel to races. I can't imagine traveling without having a race to do." Sandy Folzer explores when she travels: "Running has made travel more adventurous. When I was in Kenya with a friend and wanted to run, a Masai warrior guarded me from lions with a spear while I ran around a field. Sounds surreal and it was. When I was in Indonesia last January, I found it difficult running in the city. Being in a mostly Muslim country, I also didn't want to offend. Then, I learned that Muslim women would run in covering and only on Sunday. In Bali, which is Hindu, I ran a two-mile loop, passing nine Hindu temples, as well as rice fields."

Another rewarding consequence of running is involving family. Katherine Beiers reports: "Ten of my family members just ran a 5K/10K event, and four of us were on the podium receiving awards! One grandson won the 18-to-21 age division, a granddaughter placed in the 5K, and my 51-year-old son and I won our age groups. My son is an excellent runner. We usually do marathons together; he always runs Boston when I do—an hour and a half ahead of me, and he's at the end cheering me in. That my family members are runners makes me very proud. It's really wonderful." Jackie Yost says, "We have three children and two grandchildren. The children, now in their 50s, and the grandchildren, in their 20s, are all triathletes. We're very, very proud of that fact. We've passed it on."

With regard to food, a few women profiled pay no attention to diet, but most tend to eat balanced meals, preferring fresh fruit, vegetables, whole grains, yogurt, fish, and poultry, while avoiding or limiting red meat, sweets, or processed foods. A few are vegan. Calcium and glucosamine/chondroitin are the most commonly used supplements. Some, but not all, use sports drinks and energy supplements.

The advice they'd give to new runners can be summarized as follows: Buy good shoes at a local running store where you can support your running community, get the specialized help you need to choose shoes properly, and ask all your running-related questions. Join a running club and ask even more questions. Running stores and clubs present opportunities to participate in group runs and for socializing. Start slowly by running, then walking intervals "post to post" as one woman put it. Enjoy it. Start to race as soon as you can run three miles without stopping. Don't worry about your speed.

I hope these stories will be more than motivating. Ideally, they'll provide readers with new training ideas, new goals, ideas for good nutrition, and ways to deal with injuries. They're presented in chapters divided by the five-year age groups generally used in long-distance races.

CAROLE O. DONOHUE
March 15, 2012

Cape May Court House, New Jersey

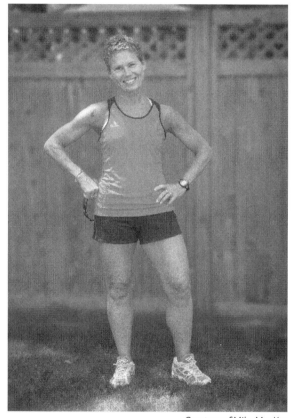

Courtesy of Mike MacKay

Age: 51

Started running: Age 29

Current training per week: 40–60 miles (training for marathon)

Long run: 8 miles off-season and up to 24–30 if training for a marathon or ultra-marathon

Best race: St. George Marathon, Utah, at age 44, 3:20

When I turned 50 I thought, "What could be more appropriate than to run a 50-mile ultra?" I applied to do the JFK 50, a large, prestigious, difficult race for which you have to qualify. I used my marathon time. The course includes 14 miles of single track on the Appalachian trail with lots of rocks. I was 10th in my age group.

Early Years and Family

I was born in Buffalo, New York, and moved with my mom and little sister to Sarasota, Florida, at the age of 13. My parents were separated. My mom was Scottish/English with a little bit of Cherokee. My father was Irish and German. Both my parents were physically fit. My father was a natural athlete who played basketball in college and squash into his 70s. My mom played tennis, practiced yoga, and walked the beach. I feel blessed that I have such good genes and wonderful role models.

Although I loved the outdoors I wasn't involved in organized sports in school. I was more of a "hippie," hanging out. I played tennis for fun, not competitively. I was a lifeguard for a while. I loved to swim, but again, not competitively.

I met my husband when I was 19 and we married seven years later. We had our 25th wedding anniversary last year. My husband was a surfer. He began to run about seven years ago. I wanted him as a pal to run and to race with. He started doing 5Ks, then triathlons. Our 14-year-old daughter has the perfect runner's body and is part of the high-school track and field team this year! She's not really excited about it, but the bug might bite!! She has the genes. My husband's second cousin is Erin Donohue, who qualified for the U.S. team at the 2008 summer Olympics in the 1500 meters.

Getting Started

In Sarasota I became a gym rat for a while. I was at the gym two hours a day, five to six days a week for fitness: an aerobics class for an hour and then the weight machines for another hour. Eventually I got tired of being inside, so I decided I would start running. One night after work I went out to run a mile on the sidewalk. And I tripped!! Sidewalks are awful for running because they are so uneven. I never ran on sidewalks again. I cut back on the gym and substituted running for half the workout.

There were a couple women at my gym who wanted me to go out and run with them. I refused because I didn't think I was good enough. I began running in June, turned 30 in July, and started racing one-mile fun runs in September.

In Florida, September is the start of the racing season. I progressed to 5Ks and five-milers and, after three years, I did the Gasparilla 15K in Tampa. Back then that was my marathon. I joined the Manasota Track Club, which was based in Sarasota, and really liked it. I found then that running was a great way to meet people with similar values. Everyone was so friendly.

Progression

After a while I started winning the one-mile fun runs—the first woman overall. I was the female winner of a race called Run and Lift. You ran a mile, bench-pressed 40-pound weights (10 reps), and ran another mile. My first award was a beach towel with the name of the race. It is threadbare and I want to throw it away, but my husband won't let me.

We moved to New Jersey in 1998, a year after our daughter was born. My first marathon was Marine Corps in 2000. I picked Marine Corps because it is "the people's marathon." No elite runners, no money prizes, just an all-American race. To train, I followed advice from veteran marathoner friends in combination with a 20-week program that I copied from a magazine. I did it on my own, just stuck to it. Eleven family members, including my husband, son, and daughter, went to Washington with me. I wanted to run under four hours. Toward the end everything was hurting—it was so hard. I was crying when I saw my sister and brother-in-law in the park as I was going up the last hill. My time was 3:59! I was hooked.

I then ran the Ocean Drive Marathon in New Jersey the next spring and the Dublin Marathon in the fall. I picked Dublin so I could connect with my Irish heritage. Since then I have run the Philadelphia Marathon twice; the Chicago marathon twice; Steamboat Springs, Colorado, with my brother running his first marathon; Steamtown in Pennsylvania; the Wine Glass Marathon in Corning, New York; the St. George, Utah, Marathon; the Las Vegas, Sarasota, and Rome (Italy) marathons; the Baltimore Marathon twice; the Atlantic City marathon; the Richmond, Virginia, Marathon; and the Ocean Drive Marathon two more times. I also did the Long Branch, New Jersey, Marathon with Dean Karnazes, his 49th of 50 marathons in 50 days!!! (See *50/50: Secrets I Learned Running 50 Marathons in 50 Days—and How You Too Can Achieve Super Endurance!* by Dean Karnazes. Grand Central Publishing, August 12, 2009.) My favorite year of racing was 2003: Rome in March, Chicago in October, and then the New York City Marathon just two weeks later.

I've gone to Boston six times consecutively, requalifying every year. I'm kind of obsessively committed to Boston now. It's a great race, although running with the crowds throughout the race is tough. But the volunteers and the cheering spectators motivate you to keep going. I raised over $8,000 running for Memorial Sloan Kettering Cancer Center and for pediatric cancer research (Fred's Team) in Dublin and in Rome, as well as in the New York City Marathon. I ran the Deadwood Half Marathon in South Dakota—a beautiful course—and would like to do the full marathon. I like to travel and race, so I pick marathons partly on the basis of the destination. I run two to four marathons a year.

After about three years of running marathons, I thought I needed another challenge to get out of my comfort zone. A friend lent me a bike to do the Stone Harbor Triathlon, a sprint. I liked it. So I did another with the borrowed bike and then I bought my own bike. Unfortunately, I started racing too much. I was doing three triathlons a month from May to September. I enjoyed the tris, but although I was placing in my age group at times, I didn't feel I was getting all I could out of it. Even though I was sticking to the sprint distance, the training was hard; the races were supposed to be the reward for all my hard training, but they got to be too time-consuming and it began to feel like a job. So about a year ago, after eight years, I stopped doing tris.

I ran my first ultra in 2010. I turned 50 in July and thought, "What could be more appropriate than to run a 50-mile ultra?" I applied to do the JFK 50 in Boonsboro, Maryland, in November. The JFK is a large, prestigious, difficult race for which you have to qualify using a 50K, 50-mile, or marathon time. I used my marathon time. The course includes 14 miles of single track on the Appalachian trail with lots of rocks. My time was 10 hours, 40 minutes—10th in my age group, and 115th out of 231 women finishers. Now I know what I need to work on: strength training for my ankles, calves, and hamstrings—so I'll do one-leg lifts. My nutrition was perfect. I used Perpetuem® powder (a Hammer Nutrition® product), which you can mix with water at any strength. I used three times the standard strength in water that I carried with me. Each dose lasted three hours. I wore my hydration pack, trail-running shoes, and gaiters to keep stones and other debris from getting in my shoes.

Injuries

Until last summer I had experienced only minimal injuries. I've had plantar fasciitis, a pulled hamstring, and sciatica. I was out six weeks with plantar fasciitis. What finally cured it was the active release technique: scraping the sole of my foot to break up the scar tissue. In the JFK race, I twisted my ankle twice and dislocated my pinkie. Now I have been sidelined with Achilles tendonitis for five months. I never thought that running defined me, but when I lost the ability to run, I found out that it does. So, to get my endorphins flowing freely again, I took up biking. I did my first century ride in the fall of 2011, the Belleplain Fall Century, a full 100 miles. Often, when I couldn't run, I went to the gym for spinning or cardio core.

Last summer I started experimenting with minimalist shoes. I was up to running in them two days in a row for six and a half miles after having them for only a month. My vision was to run more naturally—like a child. It felt very different from running in my usual shoes. I felt some strains in my foot so I was careful. Unfortunately, these shoes were NOT RIGHT FOR ME. The lack of support caused a terrible injury for which I had to seek out loads of medical advice from acupuncturists, podiatrists, sports orthopedists, and physical therapists. It took six months before I was back on track.

I see a chiropractor every other week for an adjustment when I'm training for a marathon or ultras. My chiropractor also scrapes my feet, sometimes my hamstring. I try to get a massage every three weeks. I will be running my seventh Boston in April of 2012!!!

Finding Time

When I had my daughter, I decided I wasn't going back to my nine-to-five job. Now I work as a server in a fine-dining restaurant in Avalon, New Jersey, in the summer. I like the job because I love people. And it's physical—you don't just stand or just sit. I have more time to train.

My daughter was two to three years old when I started marathoning. I loved my baby jogger, especially because when I ran without the jogger, running was a breeze. I started exercising and then running so I could be physically fit—strong and independent. I got up very early to train while she was still sleeping, then made her breakfast when I got home. My husband and my son, who is nine years older than his sister, were very supportive and helped out. I usually did my long runs on the weekends.

Diet

As far as my diet, I eat whole grains, turkey and chicken, and red meat about once a week. I love tuna and sushi, Greek yogurt, breads and tapenades, nuts, fresh fruit, and lots of vegetables—the greener the better. We also need our treats. One very important reward from training and running long-distance is celebrating afterwards! Big burgers and beer or champagne...or a couple of margaritas—it's all good. People think that because I run I can eat whatever I want. Not true.

I use a GNC® women's powder vitamin with lots of iron. I make a shake with whey protein, peanut butter, a banana, the vitamin powder, and ice cubes. If I can't make the shake, I mix the vitamin powder with water. I can't take vitamin pills. They make me feel nauseous. I feel my body absorbs the powder much better.

I drink only Gatorade or vitamin water if I'm at work and feel I need electrolytes. When running and sweating for more than an hour I use a Hammer Nutrition® product, Endurolytes®, which replenishes the electrolytes that I lose. I also use Hammer HEED®, a carbohydrate electrolyte powder that I mix with water. It's most important in hot and humid weather to replace the potassium and sodium you lose through sweat. If I'm going to be out more than an hour and a half, I know I'm going to need more than water. So I'll bring Hammer HEED® or just water and gels. I don't like to eat while I run—I feel that energy is more available in the drinks and gels. But for a training run more than 20 miles I use Perpetuem® for the protein to feed my tired muscles. Since Perpetuem® has no electrolytes, I use Endurolytes® with it.

Shoes

I've used Mizuno® stability performance shoes since my first marathon. I've tried a lot of different shoes. I put Superfeet® orthotics in my work shoes as well as my running shoes. After you wear them for about ten days they mold to your feet. They cost about $35 a pair but are well worth it. I have a sponsor in Stone Harbor, New Jersey (Global Pursuit), that will be supporting my running addiction, i.e., shoes, race entries. I will be their running billboard across America.

Helping Out

Once a week, I volunteer at the Blind Center in Avalon, New Jersey, teaching an exercise class to the blind and visually impaired. I also assist a couple of the members with their "To Do" lists. And I've been volunteering at local 5Ks. I like to help; it feels good to give back. Even though I no longer do triathlons, I still belong to the South Jersey Triathlon Club and help them support 5Ks. I'll encourage newbies, give them training tips. If people want to run, and think they can't do it, I'll tell them to take their time, start slow. Concentrate on getting your breathing under control; then look at your feet. I don't recommend wearing headphones because they make it hard for people to listen to their breathing and figure it out. I don't wear headphones because I like to be part of where I am.

Current Goals

In May and June I take off from real training. I don't do any speed work, tempos, hills, or long runs. I may go on a bike ride by myself or with my husband for fun. I'll start training in July for my fall marathons and/or ultra, then take a break in December and start training again after the first of the year for spring races. I'd like to do another ultra this spring in addition to running Boston.

In another year I may stop running Boston and concentrate on the ultras, maybe a 100-miler or a 24-hour run, where you run as far as you can in 24 hours. Last year I read about and practiced chi running. It's a method of running more elongated and with a light lean, landing on your mid- or forefoot and kicking back. No heel striking. Your elbows move back, not forward. The goal is to use your core, your lower abdominals as your gas tank. It takes a lot of concentration. Chi running holds the promise of my being able to run longer in life.

One thing I learned this past year, though, is that we don't really want to change how we run too much. You can "clean up" your stride and stature but don't go overboard and change your entire mechanics of running. Everyone has his or her own NATURAL RUNNING FORM. Be patient, listen to your body, and just make little adjustments here and there!!! Run like the wind.

In the Future

I want to be running like Joy Hampton when I'm her age. She's 14 years older than I am and we're neck-and-neck in races now...so it's not likely that I'll be able to do that. I will run until I can't. I want to run forever.

I do hope that my kids see me as a role model, as I did my parents. I'd like nothing more than to have them follow the same healthy course I do. I'd like to train them. It would be great for the whole family to go to competitions together. And then I'd like to see my children pass that lifestyle down to their children. It's about "paying it forward."

LILLIAN FELICIANO
Philadelphia, Pennsylvania

August 14, 2010

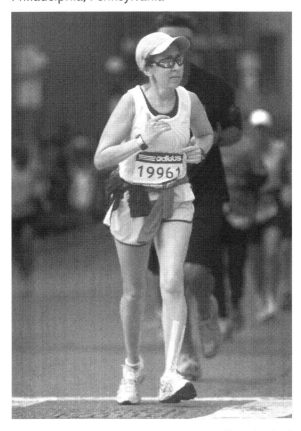

Courtesy of MarathonFoto®

Age: 51
Started running: Age 43
Current training per week: 30 miles
Long run: 14 miles
Best race: Philadelphia Marathon at age 50, 3:52:30

For a while dance was the main way I stayed in shape and maintained my flexibility. Then I tried running and liked the adrenaline rush.

Early Years and Family

I was born in Puerto Rico and moved to the New York City at age seven. The adjustment—mainly learning English in a Spanish-speaking household—was relatively easy. It took about a year to become fluent. I have two sisters and two brothers. We moved to Philadelphia in 1982 because my parents thought it would be a less hectic environment than New York. I graduated from high school in New York City and then went to Bronx Community College. I finished community college in Philadelphia and then went to Hahnemann University to become a physical therapy assistant.

Physical Education was a requirement in high school and I believe that was very good for me. It set the stage for my practicing physical fitness. Unfortunately PE is not required anymore in many high schools. Our parents encouraged us to be athletic and we all felt that it helped us do well in other areas. I took dance (modern jazz and a little ballet) at the community college, and for a while that was the main way I stayed in shape and maintained my flexibility. I took some dance courses after college and competed in *Dance Fever* in 1982, and I did some local videos and won a competition. But the cost and the rigid class schedule did not fit well with my work, and the classes were expensive. I needed something less structured.

Getting Started

I started running at 43. I had joined a gym and saw people running on treadmills. I tried it and liked the adrenaline rush. I thought, "I can do this." It became addictive. My youngest sister, Julie, is a runner. She belonged to a running group that I joined later. Basically, I wanted to stay in shape—to be fit and see how long I can stay fit.

I started by jogging a mile, and after I felt comfortable, I increased the distance to two miles. It was easy because I was already in good shape. In less than two weeks I was running three miles. I ran a couple of races but was not happy with my speed. I felt I wasn't challenging myself enough. My sister's running group did weekly speed work, so I joined. Called Peak Performance, it was a group of very mixed runners in terms of age and ability. There were 20-year-olds, 60-year-olds, and one woman in her 70s.

Progression

I went once to see what it was like, loved it, and then went every week. The workout consisted of a warm-up, running various distances from 100-meter to quarter-mile intervals as fast as you could, and then a cool-down. It took a while, but just that amount of speed work helped considerably. I saw a difference in my speed after a week or two. After my speed improved, I started doing 5Ks as hard as I could and that increased my speed greatly. My times kept improving, and I started racing a lot and getting more and more age-group medals, which was exciting. Then I cut back some on racing and started to work on the quality.

I was finding the 5Ks too short and started competing in longer races: 5-milers, 10Ks, half marathons. As time went on I wanted to challenge myself more and more. Running marathons became my goal. That's where I wanted to be. So I needed to do longer training runs. They were a little difficult. I would struggle after 10 miles or so, and was sore. To do the distances, it became more important that I eat and rest properly. You have to prepare differently than for shorter races. To run a half or full marathon, you have to maintain your speed by doing speed work once a week, a long run once a week, and other short runs and hill work once every two weeks or so. This improved both my endurance and strength.

I used to run five days a week with two days' rest. Then I figured out a way to run less, achieve the same goals, and have more rest time. Because your body really does need to rest. Now I'm running only four days a week and resting three. I'm doing longer "short" runs, one long run, and hill work, and still achieving the same fitness goals.

Injuries

I've had injuries several times, but nothing really major. Some muscle strains. The most significant was an ITB tear. This happened during the Philadelphia Marathon, my first marathon. I was 45. I ran it without being properly prepared. I was running long runs and 30 miles per week. I decided to do the marathon on a whim. I thought I could do it. Now I believe that 40 miles a week is a minimum for marathon training.

My physical training program helps me avoid injuries. I go through a regular stretch program. I know the injuries, so I know what muscle groups to work on. I know exactly how to train my body to get it back into peak shape after an injury, and to avoid reinjury.

Finding Time

Unlike a lot of runners, I do not have trouble finding the time to train. I have no children, and while I know mothers of young children who run, they have more trouble finding time. You do have to put a lot of time into training to stay at a high fitness level. My sister Julie, for example, is married and has continued to run well after the birth of her son. Her husband is also a runner and very supportive of her running—to the point that he tells her she must go out and run.

Current Goals

My current running goal is to continue to run marathons. So far, I have run the Philadelphia Marathon six times, and the next Boston will be my fifth. Going to Boston was very exciting. Boston is considered an elite marathon because the only way you can run Boston is by qualifying at another marathon. You must run a time based upon your sex and age.

I plan to run Boston every year as long as I can. I would also like to do Marine Corps and Baltimore, and to do more traveling to marathons. I would like to go back to Puerto Rico to compete in two races. One is the Best 10K in San Juan, which goes over the Teodoro Moscoso Bridge. Also well-known is the San Blas half marathon in Coamo. It is very hilly, challenging. Many elite runners do it.

I plan to continue improving in the near future. Of course, it is always nice to enter a new age group, as that provides more opportunities to place in races. I've experienced everything I wanted through running. I'm fit. I feel as strong and energetic as when I was 25. I'm slender and look much younger than my age. An unexpected bonus is all the wonderful friends I've made through running.

I try to encourage young women to start running. I've succeeded with my sister Olga, who is 48. She has lost some weight and run a few short races. I tell women who I meet in my physical therapy practice what running could do for them.

Benefits

Running has more than met my expectations. I've stayed in shape and have met some wonderful people through the years. I've traveled to races. It absolutely has decreased my stress, especially with long-distance, which I enjoy the most. My job as a physical therapy assistant can be stressful; then after I go on a short run of seven miles I feel great.

In the Future

I want to continue running all my life. At some point I will probably cut back to shorter races. Then I'd like to give back to the running community by volunteering at races. I appreciate so much what the many race volunteers do for us.

ABBY RAVEN
Treasure Island, Florida

March 6, 2011

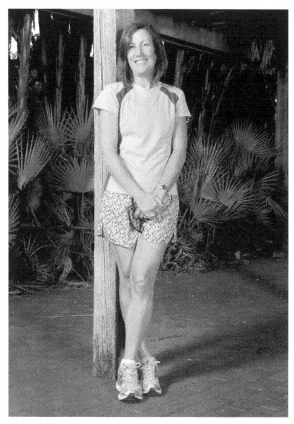

Courtesy of Mike MacKay

Age: 51
Started running: Age 39
Current training per week: Three days, 15–25 miles
Long run: 6–7 miles
Best race: Women's Half Marathon, St. Petersburg, November 2010—because I finished it!

A nice unexpected benefit of running is that I look younger than most women my age. My husband tells me that I don't look so good by accident. He knows how hard I work at it. But it is more than vanity. I'm looking for balance. I view exercise as part of a healthy life. Without it there is something missing in my life.

Early Years and Family

I grew up in Palos Verdes, California, a beautiful bedroom community right on the water south of Los Angeles. My parents were married for 52 years. My father died two years ago at 88; my mother is 86 and still in the house where we grew up. I have a younger brother.

I've exercised all my life. I was a tomboy—on the softball team in high school; I played tennis, swam, and was a junior lifeguard. I didn't want to be a boy, simply a girl who was good at sports. I was a fast runner and even good at football. The area where I grew up had the equivalent of girls' Olympics. We had uniforms, and it was very competitive. I was into that. My parents encouraged me. They never said "no" to my sports ambitions.

I didn't go to college right after high school. Instead, I started working for a rental car business at the Los Angeles airport. I was promoted quickly to a management position with significant responsibilities. I moved to the Tampa Bay area when my first husband was transferred here. We had visited for a week in April when it was glorious—sunshine and water and beautiful beaches. No one told me about the bugs and humidity in the summer.

I went to the University of South Florida (USF), originally to become a teacher, until I learned that I would have to take a huge pay cut. I was working at the time for the phone company and continued working full-time while I earned a generic social sciences degree. In 2002 I transferred to the University of Tampa for my MBA, still working full-time—and exercising. Exercise has always been a habit. I was traveling a lot too, so I was busy.

My first husband did not want children, and my second husband and I are having too much fun.

Getting Started

Where I worked, there was a gym in the basement and a group of us went there at lunchtime. A very fit coworker, Magda, got me into running in 1999. Sometimes Magda and another coworker would go outside to run rather than go to the gym. They would ask me to go with them and I kept telling them, "I'm not a runner." I finally agreed. The first time I went with them—it was lunchtime in Tampa in the hot summer sun—I was dying. They did a 2.5-mile loop. I thought, "I'll never be able to do this! It's killing me!" I went out again, though, and I finally got to the point that I could keep up. Then when fall came and it got cooler, running was easy. I suddenly realized, "I'm a runner!" A few coworkers, including my current husband and the 70-year-old father of one coworker, did Gasparilla. It was a social event—we walked/ran in over three hours.

Progression

I started registering for 5K and 10K races. I like being registered for a race because it motivates me to train. I've done the Susan G. Komen race every year; it's a zoo, too big but for a good cause.

I started running with a couple guys from work, including my current husband. There came a time, though—when I was about 45—when I realized I could not run every day. It was too hard on my body. I needed breaks from the pounding, so I did other kinds of exercises. I did not really train for races then, so it surprises me that I had some of my best Gasparilla times around that age.

I have done a few sprint triathlons. The first time I didn't train, just went to do a comfortable race. It was a fun adventure, though bike racing scares me. I hit a car once with my bike—something I'll never forget. I have a cruiser bike that I ride around my neighborhood—I love that. I'm a decent swimmer. Once in a tri I got into a fight with a girl who kept kicking me during the swim. So I haven't done a tri for a number of years. I was the runner on a tri relay team once, and that was awful because of the waiting. Now that we belong to a gym with a good pool, I may try to do some swimming again. It's great exercise.

In road races I'm mainly competing with myself. Every once in a while I'll have moments of competing with someone else in a race. It happens when someone about my age or younger, or someone who looks less fit than I am, is close to me in a race. A few years ago at a 10K a woman was on my shoulder for nearly the whole race—maybe drafting—then near the end we were even and I decided not to let her beat me. So I basically sprinted the last quarter mile. She knew and picked it up, but I outkicked her. It was ugly. I was totally spent when I crossed the finish line. I went up to her afterwards and apologized—I don't know what got into me.

Sometimes at a big race like the Gasparilla 15K, I'll kick at the end—makes for some really bad pictures. I pace myself now, so that I always have something left. I've learned not to go out too fast. Although I don't keep an organized log of my races, when training for a particular race like the Women's Half Marathon, I'll note distances completed each day on the calendar. I've recorded my Gasparilla times since 2003. 2004 and 2005 were my best times: 1:26:14 and 1:27 when I was 45 and 46; this year I ran 1:29 and a few seconds so I'm pretty consistent. My training in my late 40s consisted mostly of gym workouts. I did not run high mileage—maybe a nine-miler before Gasparilla. I prefer shorter distances. 10K is my favorite. I consider myself an average runner. I'm usually in the top third in my age group but don't place. I'm comfortable with that. What really motivates me is to keep running and not get hurt.

I've subscribed to *Runner's World* for about eight years and find some of the articles inspiring. My favorite is the monthly "I'm a Runner" article. I don't like the training schedules because they seem too extreme for me. I use them but with my own modifications. I would be really tired if I ran five days a week. I like the variety in my current exercise schedule. I have less soreness.

I'm much more focused and committed than before I started running. I'm faster and stronger overall. I am a competitive person by nature, and mostly with myself, so the evolution to my current running routine has been just right for me.

Injuries

I love to rollerblade but hadn't been doing it much anymore, because there are not any places near where I live that are safe for rollerblading. I once broke my elbow rollerblading, and then four years ago I broke my shoulder in a fall. I have a metal plate in it, but fortunately I've been able to get my full range of motion back. I've never had a running injury and don't want to get injured again, because I know how debilitating it is to sit around for six weeks. Sleeping was hard. I started to walk an hour a day with my arm in a sling. Then I went to a pool and let my arm float, because I knew that would be good for it. Later, I did intensive physical therapy. Just recently I skated an 11-mile loop at a park with a good skating surface. It was a great workout and I wasn't apprehensive at all. My husband had started cycling there after work while I was running a three-mile loop. But it was really too hot to run on the black asphalt in the late afternoon, so I decided to break out my skates. I plan to keep doing this, as it is great cross-training and I love to skate.

For a long time I ran in poor shoes, and my legs started to hurt when I was training for the half marathon. Some toenails turned black. So I went to a running store and was fitted with a high-end name-brand shoe. It made such a difference. The $30 or so extra cost was well worth it.

Finding Time

My training was not really structured until 2010. My current routine is affected by my work schedule and how much stress I have at work. My job as a telecommunications product manager is demanding. It's high-pressure and competitive. When I'm very busy at work, it is hard to find the time to exercise. But exercise is also necessary to reduce the stress. I know that if I wear myself out during the day, I'll sleep at night. When I have the luxury of a good work/life balance, I'll work out at the gym Mondays and Wednesdays, doing 50 minutes on the elliptical at a level 7 or 8. I try to burn 500 calories. Then I'll do crunches, stretch, and maybe lift weights one of the two days. I use light weights of five to ten pounds so as not to hurt my shoulder that I broke. In the winter, on Tuesdays and Thursdays, I run on the treadmill for 45 minutes at the gym. Now I try to leave work about 5 p.m. and go directly to the gym; however, I'm going back to a workplace that has a gym onsite so I expect to change back to a lunch routine. I always like to take Friday off. Saturday my husband and I will go to the gym together; I'll do the elliptical machine with the arm pulls because it gets my heart rate up higher. Occasionally I'll ride the exercise bike but I find that boring. I always run outside on Sundays, often on the hard, packed part of the beach. I try to get my husband to run with me—he's a cyclist trying to get back into running. With the switch to daylight saving time I may start running outdoors in the evenings on Tuesdays and Thursdays also. But mostly I train by myself. I do some of my best thinking then. I have an iPod that I use sometimes—especially in a long race like Gasparilla where the last mile is rough. A good song can take my mind off the pain in my legs. Mostly, though, I just like being outside listening to the sounds of nature—the birds were very happy today after the rain. I want to be able to hear cars too.

Diet

I was once a practicing vegetarian. Now I eat eggs, fish, and poultry, but never red meat or pork. I often eat veggie burgers when my husband has steak or pork chops. We eat a lot of beans and I try to eat only whole grains. Breakfast is usually oatmeal; lunch is yogurt or cottage cheese and fruit. We try not to eat too much snack food. But everyone has their weak moments. We had pizza last night. It's all about balance. The majority of the time you eat right; sometimes you don't. The older I get, the more I have to exercise and the less I can eat to maintain my weight. If my six-day-a-week schedule slips because of work commitments I have to eat a lot less. I take calcium for my bones along with Vitamin E and CoQ10.

Current Goals

My goal now is to keep fit and uninjured, and to maintain my current weight. I want to go as far as I can without injury. The cross-training helps. I stretch a little and was going to a yoga class once a week until I was training for the half marathon. I like people a little bit more when I know they are runners. I'm probably the most dedicated runner in my social group. I've never belonged to running clubs.

Benefits

I like the social side of running, but fitness is the most important aspect for me. Besides, I love to run. It feels good. I like being outside. I don't like running inside as much—it's a necessary evil.

A nice unexpected benefit of running is that I look younger than most women my age. My husband tells me that I don't look so good by accident. He knows how hard I work at it. But it is more than vanity. I'm looking for balance. I view exercise as part of a healthy life. Without it, there is something missing in my life. It makes me fitter and I look better, but even without these benefits, I would still do it because it makes me feel good.

My excellent overall health is another unexpected benefit of running; also my energy level is better than when I was 25. I'm almost never ill; my worst health problem was that I had a very difficult menopause—intense hot flashes and night sweats. Hormone replacement therapy was a miracle cure. And the hormones protect my bones.

In the Future

My husband and I often discuss how to find work/life balance. We hope to work only ten more years to find ourselves in a financial situation where we will have a comfortable retirement.

I plan to keep running and competing until it hurts and I have to stop. I expect I'll run about the same in five years as now, and in 10 years slower. I hope I'm still running in 15, 20, and 30 years. It's hard for me to visualize now. If I can't run I'll walk. I love to walk. I hope to cope with changes through the years by rolling with the punches and having realistic expectations.

SUSAN REICH
Ocean City, New Jersey

October 5, 2010

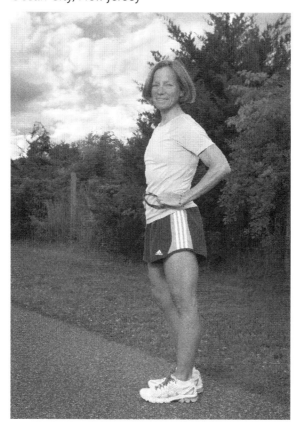

Courtesy of Mike MacKay

Age: 52

Started running: Age 22

Current training per week: 25–30 miles running, 20 miles biking, 2 miles swimming

Long run: 10 miles

Best race: Broad Street Run (10 miles) at age 49, 1:01:20

Two days before this interview Susan was the overall female winner and fifth overall in a field of 325 at the Ocean City (NJ) Half Marathon. Her time was 1:27:05, a 6:39 pace.

Early Years and Family

I was born in Philadelphia and grew up in the Philadelphia suburb of Media, Pennsylvania. My father was a structural engineer. I have two brothers and a sister. We were raised as swimmers and participated in a local swim team my dad coached. He was a swimmer and a competitive oarsman. My mom was less athletic herself but very supportive. She drove us to practices and took her turn helping out. Swimming was a summer activity that we all looked forward to. Both my brothers still swim and one is a triathlete. They come to the shore a couple times a year to compete in ocean races with me.

I went to an all-girl high school that did not have a swimming program, so I swam for a local Y Team. We practiced three times a week and went to meets on weekends, but were not at the level of the very competitive high-school teams that practiced much more. I went to college at the University of Pittsburgh and swam on the team there.

After college I went to the New Jersey shore for the summer and applied for a job on the Beach Patrol in Brigantine. One of the tests we had to pass was to run about a mile and a half under 12 minutes. I just made it in 11:50 something. When I showed up I did not know running was part of the test. I was a certified lifeguard and swimming instructor. I did fine in the swimming part, but was not prepared for the running and rowing test. I just barely made it.

Getting Started

After I got the Beach Patrol job I started running. I was burnt out as a swimmer, but still eating like I was swimming competitively, and I was gaining weight. So weight control was a motivator. In the fall I went back home and just ran casually, sometimes with our dog, so my clothes would fit. As the summer approached I started running more so I could pass the 12-minute test. And I did. Some of the girls on the Beach Patrol would go out and run during breaks, so I went with them.

I met my husband on the Beach Patrol and ran with him. He was the one who inspired me to enter my first race. We ran a 5K in the fall on the Atlantic City Boardwalk—neither of us can remember the name now or my time. I finished. At that point I ran sporadically, two or three days a week. A 5K seemed hard. I was a fair-weather runner and stopped when the weather turned cold. Then one year I ran through the winter and ran the Beach Patrol test much faster. People looked at me: "What did you do?" I said, "I didn't take the winter off."

The city Beach Patrols competed against each other in organized swims. They would send their top few swimmers. At that time there were no separate races for women so I competed with the men. I was the second-fastest swimmer in our Patrol and finished in the middle of the pack in the races. My brothers and father would come to the shore for one-mile swimming races. Then one weekend I went with a group from the Beach Patrol to a run/swim biathlon. I knew I'd do okay in the swimming, and my goal for the run was not to come in last. Actually I did very well, placing third overall.

Progression

That made a change. I was inspired to run more. Swimming is a seasonal sport in New Jersey. I would only do open-water races and they were over by September. So I kept running through the winter. I started competing more in running. The numbers grew over the years. There were certain races that I went to with friends every year. There was no specific time when I decided to be a serious runner. I didn't keep a log of my runs then, but I do now.

I work in the information technology department of a casino in Atlantic City. When I started I was working nights, so I would run during the day to fill the time. I moved to the New Jersey shore in 1984 and then to Ocean City a few years later when I got married. My husband and I rarely trained together because we had different schedules, but we did go to races together. He was the faster runner at first. Not now. He had knee problems a few years ago and had to give up running, but he still works out regularly by swimming and using the elliptical machine at the gym.

I now run early—about 6 o'clock in the morning on the Ocean City boardwalk. There's a decent crowd out there in the morning. And it is safe. It took me a while before I ran in large races. For example, in the St. Patty's Day Race that has a 5K and 10-miler, I ran the 5K for years. Looking back, I wish I had run the longer, larger races sooner. That would have inspired me to do longer training runs. I've never run a marathon. The longest race I've done is the half. As I'm finishing the half, I know I really do not want to do it again right away. The closest I've gotten to a marathon is running with friends who are training for one. If I'm going to do a long race I'd rather do a triathlon.

In the summer almost every town on the coast has a sprint triathlon, so they are close and easy to get to. I've been the first female in some. I've also been first masters woman and first female in road races. Once I was first overall in a small race. That felt good.

Training Schedule

I've cross-trained consistently. The bike is my weakest leg in a triathlon. I don't give it as much time as running or swimming. When it gets cold outside I stop biking first. I replace biking with aerobics classes, using an exercise bike, weights, and lately spinning classes, which I like. So I have not been really consistent with my bike training. In the summer I regularly do 25-mile bike training rides—out before 6 a.m. and back a little after 7. Most days I'll exercise before and after work. I don't have a long enough period of time to do it all at once. The Boardwalk is dark in the morning and evening during the winter, but it is lit so it does not matter when you run there. I go to the community fitness center to swim, row, bike, and take classes.

There aren't any running clubs near where I live. I wish there were. I like the Ocean City "fun runs"— organized, timed runs for anyone of any ability who shows up on Thursday nights at the local high- school track—which are as close to a running club that exists here. I hear about clubs in other cities and they sound great, a good way for runners of all levels to meet and train together. We have some informal groups here, but more organization would be good.

Now I mostly do shorter races, not many half marathons. I like the Olympic distance tris but there are not many around. I have never done a half triathlon and I do not aspire to be an Ironman or to go to Kona. It's too long a race. I've watched it on television and it is even long to watch.

Injuries

I've not been bothered much with injuries. I was real healthy until just before I turned 50 and got plantar fasciitis. I stopped running for two months and did cross-training including spinning. I did not lose a lot. Last year I slipped on a wet kitchen floor and landed on my tailbone. That took me out for a month. Then this summer I had Achilles tendonitis and missed most of the very active racing season. I couldn't do any triathlons this year. I did nonimpact activities like biking and swimming to keep my heart rate up and my weight down. I'm not too patient and I kept going out to try to run. I'm fortunate in that I've never had serious injuries with a long recovery time.

I do some volunteering in races now. When I'm hurt and can't run I'll go to the races and help out. I especially like to support events in Ocean City.

Fees and Costs

In order to do some triathlons you have to commit as much as six months in advance and they are expensive, $150 or more. So you can lose that money if you get injured. Some races allow you to defer to the next year or have a process for full or partial refunds if requested by certain dates, but that is only a partial solution. It is sad when there are people who want to do the race and are shut out while there are others signed up who cannot race.

Racing fees are a barrier to some people and that is unfortunate. They can add up. 5Ks can now be $40. But people are willing to pay them. Many races sell out right after registration opens.

Diet

I don't have any special diet. I can gain weight easily, so I have to watch what I eat. When I tell people that, they look at me sideways. But it is true. I try to have a balanced diet with lots of fruits and vegetables. Since I like those foods it is not difficult. I also like ice cream. I don't use energy drinks or supplements, although I have a lot of friends who do, and could probably use them in longer races. I show up with just a bottle of water. I've never taken a gel.

Current Goals

I do not have one particular goal right now. There is an annual pattern. I'll race constantly in the summer when so many races are available. The races are my speed work. I might aim for one big race like Broad Street. Then racing tapers in the fall, and in the winter I maintain my exercise routine as much as possible. This is when a running club would be particularly useful for speed work. I do not focus on one or two big races a year, but try to stay in shape so I can do whatever comes along at the drop of a hat.

I believe a large part of my success is due to my consistency. Probably good genes help. My cross-training activities all feed into my running. Slowing down some in the winter probably also helps. I don't subscribe to running magazines or read a lot about running. Sometimes I'll read an article, but basically I'm a "just get out there and do it" kind of person. I learn a lot from friends.

Benefits

I consider the fees equivalent to the cost of socializing and entertainment. We stay home a lot and do not spend money on going out to dinner and shows. Running and racing are my social life. That is where my friends are. There are women who I see regularly at races. We hang out together waiting for the awards. It's good fun. When I first started, and because running is something you mostly do alone, I did not know how great the social aspects would be. You meet all different types of people, of all ages from 70-year-olds to high-school kids, and of all different abilities. It's wonderful to see people come out and just do it. They've all accomplished something.

What do I enjoy about running? First, it gets me outside in the fresh air. Running is calming and relieves stress. I cannot run on a treadmill. I like the friends I've met. I like the muscle tone and being able to eat without gaining weight. That I've done well has been encouraging. I don't get as excited as some people about advancing to a new age group, although turning 50 was a big deal. I'm just glad to be able to still get out there and do it.

In the Future

As long as I'm having fun and staying healthy I'll keep running. I missed all aspects this summer when I was injured. I'm addicted. I think part of the reason I keep improving is that I did not start running seriously until later in life. I had much room for improvement.

CAROL ARDELL
St. Petersburg, Florida

March 2, 2011

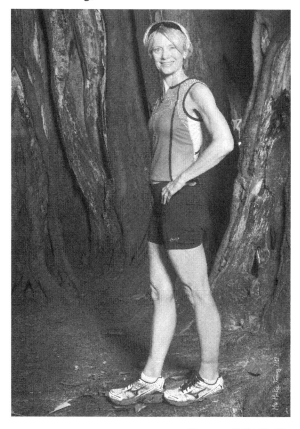

Courtesy of Mike MacKay

Age: 55

Started running: Age 41

Current training per week: 10–15 miles running, plus swimming two days and biking two days

Long run: 10 miles

Best race: Montreal Half Ironman when I was first in my age group

My husband, Don, is a huge inspiration to me, as are all the people who get up early and participate in runs/walks/triathlons, etc. I love events that bring people together in healthy and fun activities. Traveling is one of the best aspects of this sport; we travel to races. I can't imagine travel-ing without having a race to do.

Early Years and Family

I was born in Monterey, California. My dad was in the army, so we moved around a lot (army brat). I went to high school in Seoul, Korea. I felt sad about leaving my friends, but I've learned that you can make friends wherever you go. Now, thanks to Facebook, I'm reconnecting with some of my high-school friends from Seoul. This year I'm going to Beijing for the World Triathlon Championships, and then to Seoul for a couple of days to see high-school friends who remained and are working there.

My dad was the military attaché to Afghanistan in the mid-1970s, so I had an unique opportunity to see that part of the world. I come from a family of three girls. I'm the oldest. My mom is 77 and my dad is 80—both in great shape. My mom did some running for a few years and participated in several 5Ks and 10Ks. Now she goes to the gym and walks regularly. I enjoy participating in events with my family—last year my mom, my daughter, and my daughter-in-law ran a women's 5K in downtown St. Petersburg.

I did not participate in sports much until I started running and doing triath-lons. We were always active kids, learned to swim and bowl—that sort of thing. I did gymnastics in grade school and competitively in my freshman year of high school, and then was a cheerleader for several years.

My former husband and I had three children: Chris (32), Sarah (31), and Jesse (30). I have three grandchildren, with another due in July. Chris has done some running and is now into triathlons. He went to Tuscaloosa, Alabama, with us last summer and qualified for the Worlds in the sprint triathlon distance. We are going to Beijing together. Jesse has run some and my eight-year-old grand-daughter, Madison, has done the Meek and Mighty (a small tri) and will be walking a 5K with me next Saturday at the Tampa Zoo. My daughter, Sarah, will do her first triathlon this spring (Meek and Mighty). I'm very excited about that.

My first husband and I had a business. When we divorced he kept the busi-ness and I went back to school to get an MBA. I wasn't sure what I wanted to do and tried sales. I liked it but was not very good at first. So I took classes and studied with a group for eight years, and stuck with it. One reason is that I worked for a company that sold personality assessments used in hiring and, according to the assessment, I should be good at sales. I was laid off several years ago during a downturn in the economy and was out of work for a year (enjoyed it). I wish I'd known how long I was going to be unemployed, because then I could have set a goal such as doing an Ironman. In reality, I found that the more time I had to exercise the less I did.

I'm now married to Don Ardell, a pioneer in wellness. I met him when I was working on my master's degree and was doing research on wellness. I was living in Tampa and discovered that there was a wellness expert in Orlando. So I bought a couple of his books and then interviewed him. I had just started running. Don introduced me to triathlons.

I'm currently a sales and marketing professional. A person I worked with in my first job after graduate school in 1996 became the president of the company, which had moved to downtown St. Petersburg. He is now my boss and a triathlete too!! I work about 30 hours a week and have a lot of flexibility. We live in downtown St. Petersburg so I can walk to work. It's perfect. I don't have a problem finding time to train because of my flexible work schedule.

Getting Started

I quit smoking after 19 years in 1991. That was major. I felt I needed to do something to keep my mind off smoking, to relieve the stress and to feel better, so I started rollerblading. Another major lifestyle change is that I stopped drinking alcohol. The problem was that I loved wine and could not stop after one or two glasses. I wanted to drink the whole bottle. After several years I started walking with friends around a track—about three miles—in the very early mornings before I had to get my kids up for school. Some days when nobody showed up, I'd do a little running to get the three miles finished faster. I had always dreamed one day of doing the Gasparilla 15K, and decided to set that as a goal. I started running in 1996 at the age of 41. My youngest sister, Donna, was running at the time and encouraged me. She ran my first race with me, the Hidden River 10K, which I finished in just under an hour. I did my first Gasparilla in 1996. I went from jogging to racing to competing in triathlons in less than two years.

Progression/Training Schedule

My husband, Don, is a huge inspiration to me, as are all the people who get up early and participate in runs/walks/triathlons, etc. I love events that bring people together in healthy and fun activities. Don is an accomplished triathlete and runner. In triathlons, running is his strongest sport. He wins with his running speed. He won his age group in the Sprint World Triathlon Championships (USAT) two years in a row. Last year we went to Budapest; the year before that the Gold Coast in Australia for the Worlds. We usually compete in the Olympic distance but are switching to the sprint distance. We go to international competitions depending on the location, and also to events in the United States. Don is not going to Beijing, since he's not interested in traveling to China. Traveling is one of the best aspects of this sport; we travel to races. I can't imagine traveling without having a race to do.

I log my training runs (as well as swimming and biking) on a calendar. What is important is having a goal race. A specific training schedule with distances follows from the goal. We typically swim two days a week, bike two days a week, run two days a week, and rest one day. We follow one of the bike rides with a short run. The distances and intensity depend on the goal. For example, I followed a rigorous 16-week schedule for the Montreal Half Ironman when I was in my early 50s. And I had fun in the race. I'm always trying to improve, and thinking that there is a way. This keeps me motivated more than placing in my age group. I've seen a lot of people excel who started running at about the same age as I did. A lot has to do with just putting the time in. And not getting injured.

Now I am more of a triathlete than a runner. So swimming and biking are as important to me as running. There is so much to learn. Becoming a good swimmer is all about learning technique. When we first started, we went to a masters swim group that had a coach. A couple of times we went to swim clinics where we were videotaped and given pointers. There is always so much you can learn to improve in these sports—training, technique, diet. Don and I do much of our training together. We usually train in the mornings between seven and nine. He is a much faster runner than I am, so we'll go out together and after a warm-up he'll take off. We can bike together but I'm having a hard time keeping up with him now. We always do the swim workout together. We also go for a one- to three-mile walk in the evenings.

Editor's Note: Since 1996 Carol has been competing in road races, triathlons, and duathlons. She has competed on the USA Triathlon and Duathlon teams in world events and has placed in the top 10 in St. Anthony's Triathlon in her age group. When she was 50, she won her age group (50–54) in the Walt Disney World Triathlon and finished first in the Demi Sprint (half ironman distance race) Triathlon in Montreal, Canada, in 2008. She finished fourth in her age group in the USA Triathlon Sprint Nationals in 2010, to qualify for the US Team and compete in the Sprint World Triathlon Championships in Beijing in September 2011.

I do stretch some. I have an IT band stretch that I do regularly after running to prevent inflammation. It is quick and easy. Sometimes we follow a good stretching program, but it fades. My strength training currently consists of pushups. Every year I try to find the best way to add strength training to my schedule—but so far, I haven't done it. I also know I should do core work. I've done yoga and like it. Already training in three sports, it's hard to find time and energy to do even more exercise. The winter is great for training here, but the summers are very hot. Training in the summer heat and humidity can be very hard. I'm thinking of skipping a tri that I usually do in May because of the heat.

Injuries
Fortunately, I've had only minor injuries: a stress fracture on my foot, plantar fasciitis. The problem with having an injury is that it makes following a training schedule impossible. Missing a few weeks in a six-week schedule is difficult. Either you bag the race or you do it in less than top form.

Diet
After starting to run I expected that I would feel better generally and be able to "eat whatever I wanted." Fortunately, I enjoy healthful foods, for the most part. Breakfast is usually oatmeal, berries, and walnuts. Lunch varies—apple, peanut butter, or a tuna sandwich or salad. Dinner is mostly fish (other meats as well, but not as often), rice or pasta, a veggie or two. Soy ice cream or a cookie. We don't restrict ourselves by deciding we can't eat something. One of the benefits of exercise is that you burn the calories.

I take a multivitamin, folic acid, calcium, and vitamin E and C from time to time. I've recently read that you will feel less fatigued if you have an electrolyte drink before, during, and after exercise. Recently I have been feeling so fatigued after some hard training weeks that I have come home and taken a nap in the afternoon.

Current Goals
During the off-season for triathlons, I try to work on my running by participating in road races. I run 5Ks, 10Ks, 15Ks, and half marathons. I've only done one marathon—the Disney Marathon. I was having significant digestive problems at the time, which affected my race. I had thought I would try the marathon, and I did not fall in love with the distance. Nevertheless, I'd like to run Boston. I have a cousin, Sara, one year younger than I am, who has run Boston several times and keeps telling me, "You've got to qualify. You've got to come to

Boston." Last year I thought about trying to qualify at the Gasparilla Marathon at the end of February. I ran a half in January and that went okay. But I thought, "How could I train to do twice the distance in a month?" No way. So I didn't do it. But I still would like to qualify for Boston and run it with her sometime.

Doing my first tri was very a different experience from running a marathon. I loved it! On my calendar now I have the St. Anthony's Triathlon in St. Petersburg on May 1 and the ITU World Triathlon championships in Beijing in September. Long-term I'd like to do an Ironman Triathlon, and possibly Escape from Alcatraz. I'd love to go to Kona but I don't know if I could qualify. Injuries are the main barrier to achieving these goals.

Benefits

What was unexpected were so many joys. I am still emotional at the start of any event from seeing so many fit people competing. How cool it is that so many people worked hard enough to get there. I enjoy and am challenged by my work, and enjoy training and traveling to races with my husband. We both belong to the MAD DOGS Triathlon Club. I would advise anyone who is considering running to just do it! Start walking and then walking/running. Pick a 5K and find a training schedule online. If you can't find a friend to do it with you, do it by yourself—and you'll meet people there.

In the Future

I hope to be running as long as physically possible. Never stop. One of the nice things about also biking and swimming is that you have something to keep you fit when you have a running injury. I think that if I couldn't do anything but swim every day I could live with it. I've started to really like swimming. It doesn't beat you up—it's easy on your body and an incredible workout. There is nothing like eating after a very hard swim workout.

Postscript

During the first five or so years of my "second youth" as an athlete, my lifestyle was what I considered outstanding. However, I was to learn recently that it was illusory to believe, as I did, that I could feel great and go fast while eating whatever I wanted, given all the exercise I was doing. I no longer believe that.

My blood panel readings were nothing special, even though I was doing all the right things, or so I believed. I no longer smoked or drank any alcohol; nor do I stay up late, as I once did, dancing the night away. No, I was living sensibly, but I still was heavier than I thought conducive for optimal triathlon and running performances and my cholesterol was much too high.

Then I had an epiphany, with a little help from Bill Clinton! Well, Clinton's testimony about his plant-based diet got my attention, and reading books about preventing and reversing heart disease did the rest. I have been very much influenced by the work of Dr. Caldwell B. Esselstyn, Jr.; T. Colin Campbell; and many others who detail the remarkable benefits of a plant-based diet. And following that diet since August of 2011 has changed my entire outlook on food and many related lifestyle-quality issues.

Living a healthy lifestyle is not difficult, once the positive returns start being experienced. It's one thing to be as light as I was in high school and to have excellent cholesterol levels. The best part is that food tastes great.

For those who might be curious, my breakfast is usually oatmeal, berries, and walnuts with whole-wheat toast. Lunch varies—salads and veggie sandwiches and soups. Dinner is all manner of colorful plants, whole grain pastas or rice, several veggies, beans and the like. Whole Foods stores have great support for a plant-based lifestyle, as do the books *Forks Over Knives: The Plant-Based Way to Health* (edited by Gene Stone, The Experiment, 2011) and *The Engine 2 Diet* (Rip Esselstyn, Grand Central Life and Style, 2009). Recipes from these books are standards in our home. I encourage all athletes and everyone else to become informed about the hazards of the standard American diet and to look into the personal and environmental benefits of plant power.

NANCY L. SMITH
New Britain, Pennsylvania

June 2011

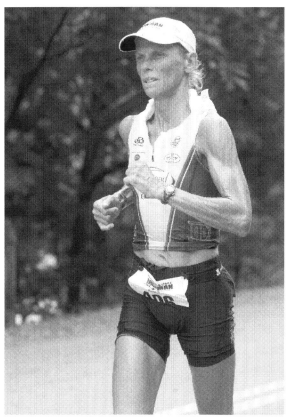

Courtesy of Brightroom, Inc.

Age: 55

Started running: Age 42

Current training per week: 30–35 miles running, 200–250 miles biking, 9–10 miles swimming (for Ironman)

Long run: 18–20 miles twice (before Ironman)

Best race: Greater Hartford Marathon at age 48, 3:14

In the past three years, my actual times—not only my age-graded scores—have improved. I believe this is due to the endurance base I have built over the years, and also genetics. In 2009 I was on the podium at Kona for the first time for being third in my age group. That was a thrill.

Early Years and Family

I was born in Abington, Pennsylvania, and grew up in nearby Huntingdon Valley. I was the only girl and went to all my two younger brothers' baseball games. I always wanted to play, but girls didn't play back then. I was on basketball and tennis teams in both high school and at Elizabethtown College in Lancaster, Pennsylvania. In high school I decided I wanted to be a physical education major in college, but my guidance counselor told me that I'd never get a job, so I decided to go for a medical secretary degree.

As I was growing up our family vacations were ski trips for one week in the winter. These were some of the best times our family had together. After I married and had children of my own, we took them on family ski trips and they also grew to love the sport.

I have four sons—ages 29, 26, 26, and 23. It was an active household. They all played golf and ice hockey. When they went off to their games, I wanted to pursue something myself, so one year we put a pool in the backyard. I swam sometimes for an hour in this little pool.

Getting Started

When we closed the pool in the winter, I felt like something valuable had been taken away, so I joined the local YMCA and started swimming laps. There I met a couple who encouraged me to try a triathlon. At the time I didn't know what a triathlon was. But I dusted off my hybrid bike and started riding to prepare. Part of a triathlon is running. I wasn't so sure I liked that part, but as I got into it, running became an outlet for me to get away for a little while. Now I love to put on a pair of running shoes and go for an hour run.

Progression

I tried a 5K shortly after starting to run, and won my age group. I have now won my age group in the Bucks County (Pennsylvania) 5K series for the past eight years. About this time (1998), I also tried my first triathlon, the sprint distance. Again, I won my age group and loved the race.

In 2002 I ran the Marine Corps Marathon, placed third in my age group, and qualified for the Boston Marathon. I also ran the Philadelphia Marathon in 2002, but I wasn't able to run Boston the next year because of an injury. I didn't run Boston until 2006, when I was training for the Lake Placid Ironman, held in New York. My Boston time was 3:46. In July I finished Ironman Lake Placid in third place for my age group, and qualified for the Ironman World

Championship in Kona, Hawaii. I have since qualified for and raced the Ironman World Championship in 2006, 2008, 2009, and 2010. I qualified for Kona at the Texas Ironman in May and am returning this year (2011). In 2009 I was on the podium at Kona for the first time for being third in my age group. That was a thrill.

I have competed in the Broad Street Run in Philadelphia for the past four years, and have placed in the top five in my age group each year, winning the age group in 2011 in a time of 1:05:37. I have run two of the races with my oldest son, Matt, and one with my youngest son, Zach. Zach is presently training for his first marathon in November 2011.

> **Editor's Note:** *Partial list of Nancy's numerous accomplishments:*
> *2002 Marine Corps Marathon, 3:27, third in age group*
> *2002 Philadelphia Marathon, 3:24*
> *2006 Boston Marathon, 3:45:29*
> *2007 USAT ranking, second in age group nationally*
> *2008 Broad Street Run (Philadelphia), first in age group*
> *2009 Ironman World Championships, Kona, Hawaii, third in age group*
> *2010 ING Philadelphia Half Marathon, 1:29:59, second in age group*
> *2010 Steelman Olympic Triathlon, first elite female*
> **Personal Bests:**
> *Marathon, 3:15 (Hartford)*
> *Half marathon, 1:25*
> *5K, 19:20*
> *10K, 40:00*
> *Sprint triathlon, 1:05*
> *Olympic triathlon, 2:20*
> *70.3 triathlon, 4:53*
> *Ironman triathlon, 10:56*

In road races I run all distances. My favorites are ten miles or half marathons. Most of the time, in local races, I have no serious competition in my age group; I'm competing against myself. In the past three years, my actual times—not only my age-graded scores—have improved. I believe this is due to the endurance base I have built over the years, and also genetics.

I am a Level 1 USAT triathlon coach. I draw up plans for people depending on their goals, abilities, and current training levels, and consult with them when they need it. The plans make training much easier for them. They just look at their scheduled workouts and that is exactly what they do. No questions, just do it and record it on their logs. It is important for me to follow my own advice, and keep a log of my training too.

I have coached many athletes, including first-timers, and enjoy seeing their progress and successes in reaching their goals. I have been a mentor for the She Rox triathlon, an all-women's tri. I also coach swimming at the YMCA, where I have been involved in running a kids' triathlon. It is fun to watch the kids getting involved at an early age and loving every minute of it. I also have coached and mentored a tri newbie class at our Y in the past.

My role models are Madonna Buder and Harriet Anderson, and athletes with disabilities—for their determination. I see people with prosthetics on one or both legs cycling on the hot lava fields in Kona. If that doesn't inspire you, I don't know what will. I also have a role model here in Doylestown, who competes with her son. Maryann Galietta, who is in her 60s, and her son Marc, who is in his 20s, compete in triathlons together. I would think that this is pretty special for the two of them. I hope one day that my son, Zach, will take up the sport and go to tris with me.

As for apparel and equipment, I ride a Guru and Trek bike and am sponsored by High Road Cycles. The staff at this store know their stuff and have spent many hours working with me to get fit properly on the bike. I buy all my running shoes from a Bucks County running store, and usually buy Asics® or Brooks® running shoes.

Injuries

Fortunately, I have not had many sports injuries. I had a stress fracture at one point, a meniscus tear another time. The meniscus tear was repaired, and I rested two weeks, then one week later I won the first race of the Bucks County 5K series. The injuries set me back in terms of racing, not training. I always had the bike or swimming to fall back on. I broke my wrist in March of 2005 and was out six to eight weeks. As soon as possible I got into the pool and started water walking and using a stationary bike. I've found that when I've been training regularly, I can take off two or three weeks without losing much conditioning. It is better to go into a race undertrained than overtrained. For a long race, tapering is very important.

I also have a team of therapists who keep me aligned and stretched, and work out any injuries that may occur. I go once every week or two for adjustments at JKM Health, managed by a local chiropractor who is also a triathlete. He works out any minor injuries or "kinks," using a variety of methods including the Graston Technique® and active release. I don't know what I would do without this help. I use the log of my workouts to write out a plan so I know how much training I need to do in any given period of time. When my arms or legs wear out in a long endurance race, I still feel that I have strength because my core is strong. I believe that these activities plus the swimming and biking are particularly important for older runners. Running is just so much harder on the body. I swim most days because it is so relaxing.

Diet

My diet consists mainly of fruit, vegetables, salads, fish, pasta, and whole grains. I cook red meat for my family. Occasionally I'll eat a little ice cream—I'd really much rather have a piece of fruit for dessert than cake or cookies. I drink smoothies that I make with a fruit-juice base, fruits in season, and sometimes a little protein powder as a recovery drink after a long workout. I take a multivitamin, and a lot of omega-3s and glucosamine that I'm convinced keep my joints lubricated. I use Cytomax® on the bike and Recoverite® after a workout. I also use gels on the bike and while running.

Current Goals

My current goal is to do well at Kona this year and possibly run a marathon in November with my son, maybe both of us qualifying for the Boston Marathon.

As I grow older I realize that I can't compete with younger women and keep the times I did. My training is not as intense and I take more rest days and enjoy them. I have been injured in the past, and from those injuries have learned that I can't swim, bike, and run 24/7. I have learned to be patient, which is very hard for a Type AA personality. To keep up with all my activity, I strength train two or three times per week, and work in yoga and stretching. I have worked with a trainer in the past who has given me great direction to help my body stay strong and flexible.

Benefits

Mostly, I love running because of the feeling it gives me to just be free and go, enjoy the break from life, the mental lift. The area where I live, Bucks County in southern Pennsylvania, is pretty any time of the year. Sometimes I'll go up to a nearby lake, be alone, pray, and listen for God. It's so peaceful. Swimming is very relaxing for me. I like to do it after a run when it feels like a massage. It loosens my legs, bringing me back into equilibrium, peace. And I like getting on my bike and just going, getting lost even. I can be out biking three or four hours. If there is such a thing as exercise addiction, I have it. I feel much better after getting out there, and worse if for some reason I can't exercise.

I would advise new runners to walk, run, walk, run until your tendons and ligaments get used to the stress. Don't increase weekly mileage too fast or you will get injured. And just enjoy the moment. Pick a trail, or go to a park and enjoy being outside. It makes you feel so alive.

In the Future

I hope that I can continue running and "triing" for many years. I have kids living in Houston, Germany, and Denver, so I have lots of places to visit and possibly do a race. I also have a grandchild on the way, so I am excited to be a grandmother.

I will continue to train by swimming, biking, and running, and competing in races as long as God is by my side and strengthening me to do this. I love being active and as long as I wake up every morning, there is somewhere new to ride and or run.

DORI ITEN
Pinellas Park, Florida

March 27, 2011

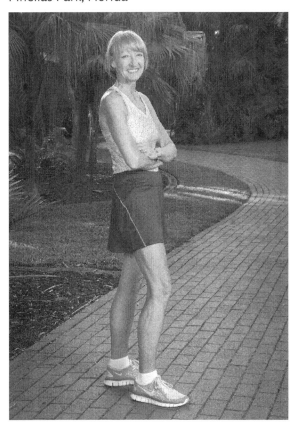

Courtesy of Mike MacKay

Age: 57
Started running: Age 31
Current training per week: 30–35 miles, 5 days
Long run: 14 miles
Best race: Rocket City Marathon (Huntsville, Alabama)
at age 48, 3:22

Once I got into running, I felt good about myself. I thought, "I'm doing something that a lot of people can't do." The self-confidence carries over to other areas of my life. And running has kept me looking more fit than nonathletic women my age.

Early Years and Family

My parents came from Germany in 1949, after the second world war. Before the war my father was a winemaker. All of their vineyards in Germany had been confiscated. In the United States my father worked as a butcher and as a janitor, and then in his 50s he bought a motel in St. Petersburg, Florida.

I was born in Dayton, Ohio, and grew up in the Chicago area, where I played baseball and softball in school. I graduated from the Evanston, Illinois Township High School, and attended Southern Illinois University for a year—something I tried to do on my own since my parents were "old school" and believed that girls didn't need college. They felt that a girl should just get married and have children. I moved back to Evanston—although my parents were in Florida by then—and worked for a while, but had no direction and felt lost.

I married at twenty and moved to Davenport, Iowa, my husband's hometown. I'm not sure why I married him. He was a heavy drinker and spent a lot of time in bars. The people in the neighborhood bar were an extended family for my husband. When I got pregnant, he did not want me to keep the baby. It was a very stressful pregnancy. I made up my mind to leave him when things did not change after the baby was born, and left when my son Dieter was a year and a half. I moved to St. Petersburg, where I worked as a word processing operator for a financial accounting firm downtown. After that, I was an administrative assistant for many years. I smoked until I was 27.

Getting Started

When I lived in downtown St. Petersburg, my son Dieter played with the son of a nearby couple who were runners. I was 31 by then and beginning to gain weight. This couple looked like they were in great shape. I tried to run by going out and running as hard as I could and lasted for about a block. That obviously wasn't going to work.

I started talking to the wife, Beth, and she said that if I wanted to start running, she would run with me and teach me how to pace myself. She ran half a mile with me the first week, then a mile the next week, and so on. She introduced me to my second husband, Ken, a very good runner. He told me that he ran 16 to 18 miles on Sundays. I couldn't fathom that. I thought he was terrific, very fit and a very handsome guy. I was in love with him. And he adored Dieter.

Then I was really motivated. I wanted Ken to like me and admire me too. I ran every day, increasing my mileage to 40 a week within a year. We ran together at times but he was much faster than I was. I ran with other runners closer to my pace, and I would support him at races.

We dated for several years. Then Dieter's father died when he was eight. I asked Ken to come with me when I told him. Dieter looked at me and said, "Who is going to be my father?" Ken stepped right up and said, "I'm going to be your dad." And he asked me to marry him the next day. Dieter was a very good soccer player and he ran track in middle school. He is now 32 years old, and started to pick up running again to stay in shape. We recently ran a 5K race together.

Progress

Ken belonged to the Forerunners Track Club. So I joined Forerunners and trained with them. Running was very competitive then. Now there are some really good runners, and then there appears to be a big drop-off to a large number of much slower runners. Twenty to 25 years ago there wasn't that same gap. It seemed like all the runners were competitive. The Forerunners coach developed a training plan for each of us. I got up to 60–65 miles per week, ran intervals, did track work—all of it. I ran seven days a week, didn't take a rest day. I can't do that anymore.

There were many fast women in my age group. I usually placed second or third, first only when the top women didn't show up. There were two faster women who were slightly older than me. When they moved into a new age group, I won everything until I moved up. Running so well meant a lot of hard work, but I was willing to do it.

I did better in longer races. I disliked the 5K distance because you had to run as fast as you possibly could from start to finish; no time for strategy. I had some good times but not great. Some women in my age group were breaking 40 minutes in the 10K. I once was the overall female winner of a local 10K with a time of 42:34—none of those faster women showed up that day!

My first marathon was Columbus, four years after I started running. I had been running half marathons and other smaller races, including the Gasparilla 15K. I've run between 25 and 30 marathons, including Boston twice. To qualify was, at one time, a major goal. Actually running Boston was a bit disappointing, since I ran well over my qualifying time. I'd hoped to do really well. I ran it in 1990, before chip timing, so a lot of time was lost getting to the starting line. Then I ran much too hard during the first part of the race trying to make up for the slow start. I was pretty well spent by the time I got to Heartbreak Hill. However, it was a thrill to have run and completed the infamous Boston Marathon.

In my 30s and 40s, training for a marathon was not hard. I always kept my long run at a minimum of 16 miles because I knew that if I dropped to shorter distances, it would be very hard to get my long run back up to 16.

I did a few ultras for a while—a few 50Ks (31 miles) and one 40-miler with my friend John, who was trying to encourage me to train for a 50-mile race. John ran the whole race with me even though he could have gone faster; with his support I finished as second female. I might have come in first, but during the last 10 miles, I became so dehydrated that my legs starting cramping and locking up. They felt bolted to the pavement at times and it took several minutes to "free them up" and get moving again.

Finding Time

Finding time to run while raising a child and working full-time was not a problem because Ken and I shared the responsibility. He'd watch Dieter while I ran and vice versa.

Several years after Ken and I divorced, I went back to school for a nursing degree. It was clear that my job in the company I was working for was not going to last, and I was concerned that I would not be able to support myself. My son was in college by then. I figured that I would always be guaranteed a job as a nurse. Since I was going to school and also working full-time, my running was put on the back burner. While it was necessary, at the same time I regretted not being able to run as I had before.

I graduated from nursing school in 2005 at the age of fifty and got my license in 2006. I took a job in a hospital with a later shift and so was able to run later in the morning. I started going regularly to a local park with nice trails to get my running back on track. I met Millie Hamilton there and started running with her regularly. After 14 months I left the hospital job for a Monday through Friday job as a utilization review nurse. While I was working at the hospital, I had to work weekends. Now I had my weekends free to enjoy the leisure activities with everyone else. Weekends are really important for runners because that is when people do long runs and that is when there are races.

I hadn't been running as much for the past two years and I'm not like some for whom running comes naturally. I have to work hard to do well, or to be in shape enough to even enjoy a run. With my current job I have trouble finding time to train. I get up at four every morning, have coffee and stretch, sometimes do a DVD abs workout or lift weights, run six miles, and then walk my dog about a mile and a half before I go to work. My dog is a small beagle mix, and he can run when he wants to, but most of the time he likes to follow his nose on some mysterious scent. I don't think it would be fair to force him to run distance. I don't do any strenuous cross-training. I have to exercise in the morning because I can't do it later. The only time I was able to run in the evening was back in the day when I was doing track after work.

I improved my fitness and started racing again. I ran the Turkey Trot 10K in 50 minutes, then the Hops Marathon in Tampa in 3:47.

Injuries

My running started to progress well until about three years ago when I developed piriformis syndrome. I'd never had an injury that was so painful and lasted so long. I tried to run through it but couldn't really extend my leg. Just walking was painful. I went out for a run on Christmas Eve, and while trying to extend my leg, my hip gave way. I landed facedown and got pretty beat up. After that, I stopped trying to run while injured, and instead walked the dog every day. I went to a physical therapist a couple of times and did some exercises he gave me. I tried the elliptical at the gym but it wasn't the same. I was "out" for six months. When I started back, I was painfully slow and very out of shape. Coming back was a struggle, like starting all over again. But I finally made it and was able to run the Philadelphia Half Marathon a year and a half ago with Millie.

Just when it seemed I was getting back to form, I developed piriformis syndrome on the other side and was "out" another four months. During that whole time my confidence was shaken and I felt less of a person than when I could run with confidence. Motivation had deserted me. In addition, last summer I began having breathing problems, almost like an asthma attack, a mile or two into a run. This was something I had never experienced before. It felt like my airways were blocked—as if I was reacting to all the allergens hanging in the humid air. I went to a doctor who suggested it might indeed be asthma triggered by some allergen and had me try a couple of different inhalers. They didn't work and I was hardly able to complete a run that whole summer. Some days I'd go out and could tell right away that I couldn't run. Other days I could run two or three miles and then my airways would shut down. I lost more fitness, became even slower—and more importantly, lost more confidence and self-esteem. I started feeling depressed when I couldn't keep up with Millie or any of our other running partners. Then the summer heat and humidity passed, giving way to cooler temperatures, and I was able to run without difficulty.

Diet

I eat a lot of vegetables, not much fruit. I love sweet potatoes; I eat chicken and fish, shrimp and some pork—all baked. I don't eat any fried foods, hamburger or other red meat or, with rare exceptions, sweets. I try to stick with whole grains. I like Greek yogurt, cheese, and pasta. Sushi is another favorite.

I take a vitamin D supplement because I've read so much about how it can boost energy. I can't really tell if it works. I've resisted taking calcium, partly because a scan showed my bone density to be great—at the top of the chart. I usually just drink water when I run. On a long run I might take a few bites of an energy bar, and on long runs on very hot days I'll have some low-calorie Gatorade®. I don't like the sweet taste of Gatorade.

Current Goals

I'm pleased that in just the last couple of weeks, my mental attitude became more positive; although I am still apprehensive about the coming summer. I've started running track again with a group and am trying to run five days a week. I find that I now want to improve, although I would have to work extremely hard to become competitive in my age group again, and that hurts. I want to become competitive again and train for another marathon. I'd like to run Boston again, but I know that would mean consistent training to qualify. And the trip to run Boston is very expensive.

Benefits

Once I got into running, I felt good about myself. I thought, "I'm doing something that a lot of people can't do." The self-confidence carries over to other areas of my life. And running has kept me looking more fit compared to non-athletic women my age. One of the unexpected benefits of running is the camaraderie. I have made many good friends in the running community.

In the Future

My goal is to stay injury-free and keep running. I'd love to be as resilient as Millie. I don't know how she trains so hard without getting hurt. I've been so plagued by injuries these past few years that I don't think about what will happen in five years or more. Ultimately, I just want to be able to run for the joy of running. I lost that feeling during the last few years when I wasn't able to run. Coming back can become a chore. I want to always be able to run. But if I can't run, I'll volunteer at races.

CAROLYN R. BUJAK
Palmyra, New Jersey

June 12, 2011

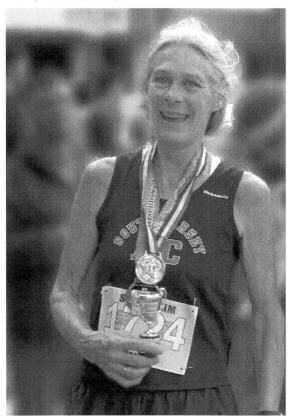

Age: 59

Started running: Age 24

Current training per week: 30–35 miles; when training for marathon, 40–45 miles

Long run: 8–12 miles; when training for marathon 22–23 miles

Best race: "Ugly Mudder" trail race at age 58

My most memorable race is the Ugly Mudder, a 7.25-mile trail run near Reading, Pennsylvania, in February 2010. We raced up and down the mountain in two feet of snow. The trails became icy, slick, deep, narrow ruts. I couldn't get a grip on anything. Good thing the snow was deeper and softer on the sides of the trail, because I spent at least half the race hauling myself out of snow banks.

Early Life and Family

One of four children born to Ruth and George Brown, I have an identical twin sister and two older brothers. We were raised in Gloucester City, New Jersey. My sister and I were the first in our family to attend college and graduate school. We were an Irish, Protestant, Republican family living in an Irish, Catholic, Democrat town. It was typical medium-sized suburbia where kids could walk everywhere. Neighbors knew neighbors and everyone else in town as well. I couldn't get away with anything.

I've been married to the same guy for 32 years. He's not a runner, but he supports my running. Our four kids, now ages 29, 26, 24, and 19, run as well. They all ran cross-country and track while in high school and continue to run and race intermittently depending upon what's happening with their college, work, and/or family schedules. So my husband is outnumbered. His stock reply to folks who ask him, "Do you run?" is "I'd rather have hot pins stuck in my eyes." His new one is "I'd rather staple a skunk to my head and attend a banjo makers' convention."

Being raised in the 1950s, I was expected to "act like a lady," sit demurely, and play with Barbie™ dolls. But I ditched Barbie whenever I could, and snuck out to find neighborhood baseball, kickball, football, stickball, or any game that involved running. In fact, I've been running ever since my mother told me not to—at about age three.

From age nine to 16, I played softball in a neighborhood league association, the Gloucester Fillies, usually in center field. My father shared coaching duties with the chief of police. On one hot, humid morning, when it was time to leave for practice, I started whining about the heat and the fact that I was "too tired" and "By the way, dad, all my friends are probably at the pool." It took my father just ten words to teach me about self-discipline in sports training. He spoke softly, "Go get your uniform; I'll hand it in for you." I got in the car.

In high school, I went from one sport to another: softball, basketball, and field hockey. We didn't have a girls' track program; it was not an acceptable girls' sport. Girls were not permitted to join the boys' team.

Inviting my children to run with me has had unexpected, unforgettable benefits. Often, running with my children provided fertile ground for the best parent/child talks. They spoke with heart-rending honesty on a run. We were on no one's turf—just outdoors, moving along together. Running freely, they spoke freely. I recall a run with my then 18-year-old daughter, a first-semester college student home for the holiday and distraught over a breakup with her high-school boyfriend. While telling her story, she began sobbing hysterically. Of course running becomes difficult when you're sobbing, so I said, "Zoe, you can't run and cry at the same time because it's hard to breathe." She stopped in the middle of the street, half-crying, half-laughing. We hugged each other, me laughing, Zoe crying and laughing, and resumed our run with a renewed spirit of moving on, moving forward.

I enjoy the private talks on our relaxed training runs together, but racing together is different. I recall playing cat-and-mouse games with two of my adult children all through the Half-Wit-Half-Marathon in Reading, Pennsylvania. We were hurling sticks and insults at each other somewhere around the nine-mile mark.

I'm currently a reference librarian at Burlington County College, Mt. Laurel (New Jersey) campus. The community-college students and faculty, along with my library colleagues, are a delightful bunch. I enjoy their company and appreciate the down-to-earth, edifying, and diverse nature of the community-college environment.

Getting Started

I began to run recreationally but steadily in graduate school (1976–1978) to clear my head, restore my soul, and strengthen my body—it proved to be a good thing. I went to the track at about 11:00 almost every night. I remember being so self-congratulatory when I achieved my personal goal of running four miles without stopping.

I was purely a recreational runner until age 45, running about two to four miles a day. One day when hiking in the New Jersey Pine Barrens, I came across an advertisement for an upcoming 10K race to be held on the sandy roads of the Pine Barrens. I loved hiking those roads and trails, so I had the audacity to sign up without a shred of racing knowledge or experience. I didn't know a soul on race day—it was a brand new game, unknown territory. I was so clueless I pinned the bottom tear tag of the race bib to my shirt—yup, the part that says, "Do Not Pin." Running this race turned out to be good intuition. I placed second in my age group, won about six pints of freshly harvested New Jersey blueberries, and met Ted and Dee Hardies of the Pineland Striders, who invited me to join their running club—I did.

Progression

The progression from jogging to racing, though, took longer than it should have. I once thought that racing was for professional or highly competitive—not "average"—runners. But later, I realized that racing provided me with the impetus to become a better runner and to train more consistently. I was curious to see if I could work my way up to a half marathon. It seemed like an incredible challenge. Race day is a little like music lesson day: You know how it will go if you skipped practice during the week.

My favorite and most memorable race is the Ugly Mudder, a 7.25-mile trail run hosted by Pretzel City Sports in Reading, Pennsylvania. This adventurous, not for the faint-of-heart race keeps me laughing from start to finish—especially the infamous February 2010 edition, when we raced up and down the mountain in two feet of snow. The trails became icy, slick, deep, narrow ruts. I couldn't get a grip on anything. Good thing the snow was deeper and softer on the sides of the trail, because I spent at least half the race hauling myself out of snow banks.

Through the years, I've learned a lot about myself and what I need to pay attention to in order to run and race well. Running and racing gets better with age. I'm getting a handle on what it takes to run a 5K, what it takes to run a marathon, what type of shoes work for me, what it feels like when I'm running really well or really poorly, and when it's time to pay attention to aches and pains. The more I run, the more I learn about running. There's no replacement for experience.

I am a member of two local running clubs, the Pineland Striders and the South Jersey Athletic Club. I race every distance from the 5K to the marathon throughout the year, averaging about 25 races a year. Most are part of the Mid-Atlantic Grand Prix, a series of both on- and off-road races prescribed by the local long-distance running committee of USA Track & Field. Racing as a team and/or club member is a hoot. The camaraderie of racing with a team elevates each runner's effort and adds greater value to the race.

Injuries

Considering the longevity of my running, I've been gifted with being almost injury-free, although occasional injuries have interrupted my training, the worst resulting in six months of no impact activity—i.e., no running. I was seven weeks away from the Philadelphia Marathon when I experienced pain and swelling behind the patella of my left knee. I couldn't walk without limping. I went to a recommended sports medicine knee specialist in hopes of a diagnosis and a quick fix, and had to wait three weeks for my initial evaluation. Two months later, following an X-ray, an ultrasound, an MRI, and a slew of strengthening exercises, my knee pain remained a mystery. I never did learn the cause of it, but I did figure out how to heal, thanks to the advice of fellow runners and pool running. I joined a gym with a pool, jumped in the deep end, and ran without a flotation device. I started with 10 minutes and worked up to 45 minutes a day over six weeks—and it worked beautifully for me.

Finding Time

Finding time to train remains a challenge. It was far more difficult when my children were young. Family, friends, work, and community commitments surround us and deserve nourishing, so I try to keep myself balanced and not become obsessed about sticking too tightly to my training schedule. My work schedule is erratic, so I remain flexible about what part of the day I run. I prefer to run as soon as I get home from work, before I get too comfortable. I run outside (no treadmill) no matter what the weather. If there's ice and snow I put ice spikes into the treads of my shoes. If it's hot and humid, I slow down and drink more water. If it's raining, well, good thing I have towels and a hair dryer at home.

As an older runner, though, I run before dark if possible; my eyesight and depth perception are not as sharp as they were. I still have a scar on my knee from an encounter with a downed tree branch lurking on the side of a dark road.

True confessions: I don't cross-train nearly as much as I know I ought to. It would probably do me good. And, racing is my speed work. Admittedly, I don't enjoy speed work. Just as with cross-training, it would no doubt be good for me, but I avoid it and substitute racing. Too much speed work and not enough play make Johnny and Sally dull runners.

Current Goals

Current goals include running the next Philadelphia Marathon in 3:29:00. A possible barrier would be my aversion to speed work and cross-training. Also, I plan to work more off-road races into my calendar.

Benefits

I ran because I discovered that it made me stronger—not just physically, but mentally and spiritually. Perhaps I'm just wired to be active and moving. I train alone. My long runs provide me with coveted private time. I can relax and hear myself think, put myself back together again—running is my reset switch. Ideas arise, inspiration appears, and decisions are made. Sometimes I make profound decisions while running, something like, "Gee, perhaps I should defrost the refrigerator tonight." Sometimes I solve deep mysteries such as, "Why is my son chronically allergic to homework and when will I find a cure?" Perceived mountains erode into molehills with each mile, and sometimes the missing piece to a puzzle is found.

Running brings a sense of place: I never get bored with my training routes. I find comfort and security in these well-worn courses. I've become one with the neighborhood. I didn't quite realize the extent of my belonging until one day when I walked the route due to a few cracked ribs. Strangers stopped me on the street and said things like, "Are you okay? Why aren't you running?" I didn't realize that I had become part of their everyday experience. I was seven miles into a 12-mile run when it started to rain heavily. Sure enough a neighbor pulled to the side of the road, waited for me to catch up, rolled the window down a couple of inches and said, "I'm guessing that you don't want a ride home, right?" It's good to be reminded that we're a small but highly significant part of something larger than ourselves.

Gratitude for the support that I've received along the way is increasingly important to my running. I'm now well aware of the tremendous work that goes into any race, no matter how small. So I find the breath to thank course marshals, police officers, folks handing out water, and all the volunteers that make the race possible.

I volunteered to assist the cross-country coach at the neighborhood high school where three of my kids ran track and cross-country. I ran with the kids almost every day and cheered them on at races. They showed commitment and courage. One student showed up at every practice, got lapped at every race, always came in last, but never quit. He did everything we asked of him without complaint. He's my hero, and I still see him around town, walking, running, or biking. We enjoy greeting each other with "Hey, slacker."

In the Future

As for my future running, I'll play the cards I'm dealt the best that I can. I expect to cope with aging by paying attention to intuition, realism, and common sense.

I cope better with changes now than when I was young, impatient, inflexible, unrealistic, and inexperienced. It takes longer to recuperate after long races now. Oh well, I've learned not to fret about it, so instead of becoming anxious as when I was in my 20s and 30s, I accept that I won't be running a 10-miler three days after a marathon. I'll chill and run a five-miler instead.

Of course, I hope to keep running and racing. I expect that at some point, my times will get slower; but that's okay, I'll make the adjustment—I doubt it will diminish my running spirit. I'm part of the Mad Runners' Liberation Front and our motto is: Run on, and on, and on.

I'm on the lookout for a T-shirt I saw on an old guy at a race about 10 years ago. The slogan read, "Growing old disgracefully," and as I remember, the guy ran well in the race, and sped off afterward in a spiffy, fire-engine-red MG Midget.

SUZANNE GIBSON

October 17, 2010

Egg Harbor Township, New Jersey

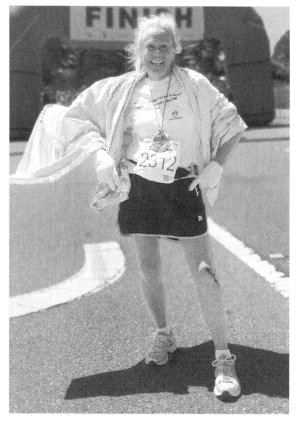

Courtesy of MarathonFoto®

Age: 60

Started running: Early 40s

Current training per week: 40 miles

Long run: At least 10 miles, 17–18 miles during marathon season

Best race: Philadelphia Marathon at age 52, 4:06

I lived in Bucks County, Pennsylvania, with easy access to paths in a beautiful state park. I attribute a lot of my development as a runner to that park. There were significant hills, shaded trails, open spaces, streams. Running alone in that place was truly glorious—a terrific way to relieve stress and find peace.

Early Years and Family

I was raised in the Philadelphia suburbs. I have two sisters and a brother. My brother, Paul, who is now 58, will race occasionally. One sister, Maureen, has tried running and liked it, but doesn't have the time right now. My other sister, Sheila, has multiple sclerosis—we're very close. I am so inspired by her. No matter how poor her health, she just keeps going and her attitude is consistently positive. I've done the city-to-shore bike ride benefiting multiple sclerosis to support her.

There were not many varsity sports available at the high school I attended in the 1960s where I was a varsity cheerleader. I attended nursing school in the late 1960s and early 1970s. Until I started running, I did not participate much in sports.

I was married and have three adult children. My partner, Michael, has three daughters. We like to consider ourselves one family with six children and five grandchildren. My oldest daughter, Suzanne Marie, has done sprint triathlons and is a member of a running club. My son, Brendan, is also a running club member and will be finishing his first marathon at the end of this month. He lives in the Philadelphia area and comes to the shore frequently in the summer to run in races with me. My youngest daughter, Brighdin, and I share our disappointment if our schedules don't permit us to fit in our runs. Although she prefers to run five miles at a time, she recently told me that she has encouraged herself to feel content with days that she can only fit in shorter runs of one to three miles. I think this would be a good lesson for all mothers of young children: that running one mile is better for you than not running or exercising at all.

My ten-year-old granddaughter, Maren, is a runner and has completed some triathlons. She is currently participating in Girls on the Run, a program that empowers young girls through both training and providing role models.

Getting Started

I started walking at a time of change in my personal life with no intention of running. I progressed by walking longer and longer distances. After a while, walking long distances became boring, so I started jogging, and then that jogging led to running. I enjoyed getting outdoors and running. I lived in Bucks County, Pennsylvania, at that time, with easy access to paths in a beautiful state park. I attribute a lot of my development as a runner to that park. There were significant hills, shaded trails, open spaces, streams. Running alone in that place was truly glorious—a terrific way to relieve stress and find peace.

I did have one role model, though. When I was in my 30s, I remember meeting the wife of my son's high-school baseball coach, Mary Weeden, a woman in her early 60s at that time. She was wearing a new New York City Marathon jacket. I asked her whose jacket it was. She seemed a bit insulted (as I now know she should have been) as she replied, "Mine." I did file the thought in my brain that day that maybe I would try to run that marathon someday! I did it in 2004.

After I had been running for years, a local man who was a runner approached me and said that he had been noticing me running around our town and in the state park, and asked me if I had ever thought about doing a race. I said no although I knew that races were out there...somewhere. He said he thought I was ready. That's how, at the age of 50, when I had never participated in any race, I found myself at the starting line of the Philadelphia Marathon. After registering for the marathon, I did call Mary and tell her what I was doing. Although she supported me, she was concerned because I had not run any races previously.

I did not tell anyone else that I was running that marathon—in part because I thought they would think it was crazy to have my first race be a marathon, and in part because if I failed, no one would know. I hadn't used a training schedule, I didn't know what my training distances were, and I had not read anything about running and racing. I did not even own proper cold-weather running clothes. I got to the start very early and parked close to the starting line. There was a gentleman parked behind me reading a newspaper. I asked him a few basic questions. The race went well, especially considering what I know now about running. My time was about 4:45. I was close to tears when I crossed that finish line, elated.

Progression

After that, I was interested in learning more about running and joined the Bucks County Road Runners. They welcomed me. It was great to see such a cross-section of the population represented in the running community. A person's profession, ethnicity, age, or ability did not matter. Everyone was accepted equally. The fast runners encouraged and supported the others.

About the time I joined the club I started picking up running books and magazines. My favorite is *Runner's World*. They had a section entitled "You know you are a runner if you"...and then it would describe a behavior characteristic of runners. One of my favorites was "You know you are a runner if you only turn on the television for the Weather Channel."

The president of the running club at that time lived close to me in New Hope, Pennsylvania. I did a lot of my running back then on the tow path along the New Hope canal, and sometimes ran with him. One day he encouraged me to run the Philadelphia Marathon again, saying that a lot of the club members would be there. Although I never intended to run another marathon, I went home that day—only a couple weeks before the race—logged on to the marathon website, and registered. Once again I would run a marathon without doing a training program.

My partner, Michael, drove me to that second Philadelphia Marathon, and intended to bicycle along and meet me about every five miles to give me water and GU. He only made it to the first five miles; his bike fell apart. At about the half marathon mark, I asked the bystanders if anyone had a GU and someone from the crowd gave me one. At about mile 20 another runner gave me my last GU. I remember feeling so comfortable. I never run with a watch, so I wasn't paying attention to my time. When I crossed the finish line I saw the runner that I had met the previous year. He greeted me excitedly, looking at the finish-line clock, and said, "I think you just qualified for Boston." He sent me the qualifying times later with a congratulatory message saying that I had just met the time requirement. The most amazing thing to me was that I had stopped several times along the course to talk to friends. I vaguely knew from listening to other members of the Running Club that Boston was a big deal, but had not paid much attention.

I had to go to Boston. And then running became not quite so much fun. I needed to train hard. Running through the winter was tough. I had to train in the dark. It was cold and lonely. I worked all day as a nurse and then ran 10 miles many nights.

I felt honored going to Boston with some of the members of the running club. But I also felt that I deserved to be there because I had done the training under difficult circumstances. Boston that year was a tremendous struggle for me. I finished in about 4:45 with only vague memories of the race. As I went across the finish line I told myself that I would never run again. But a day later I decided that I would run again, a week later I decided that I would run marathons again, and about a month later I decided I would run Boston again.

When I went back to Boston the next year, I vowed that I would enjoy the experience. The thrill of marathon morning was mixed with apprehension because of projected record high temperatures. (The temperature did reach a record high of 86 degrees.)

My daughter, Brighdin, was a student at Gettysburg College that year. She was talking with some friends the day before and said that her mother was running the Boston Marathon. One of her friends said, "If my mother was running the Boston Marathon I wouldn't be sitting here, I'd be on my way to Boston." On impulse they organized themselves, got into a van, drove through the night to Boston and went to the Wellesley College—the Wellesley College campus borders the Boston Marathon course, and the Wellesley girls are legendary for their loud screaming as the runners go by. Brighdin's good high-school friend, Ashley, a Wellesley student, knew I was running and had made a huge banner with my name on it. So there was a large group of Wellesley and Gettysburg college students, including my daughter, holding the banner at the end of the campus (which is about the halfway mark of the marathon). I stopped to talk to them until my daughter said, "Run, you can't spend any more time here."

I don't like to run 5Ks. The crowd goes out so fast. I think, with distractions such as iPods, that not everyone is safe. You risk injury. I like running races on the beach, near the water. I am also very fond of trail running. Trail running is the closest I get to feeling like a child again. Running so freely up hills and down to meadows, stream crossings, getting soaking wet, jumping over fallen trees...it's all there. The challenge is in watching your footing and also in trying to comfortably pass another runner.

About five years ago I moved from New Hope to New Jersey. I was disappointed when I discovered that there were no running clubs here. Although I am comfortable running alone for many miles, I miss the camaraderie of other runners.

Training Schedule

Now most of my training is done on the three days of the week that I have off from work. After my 10-hour shifts as a nurse I find that I am usually too tired to run. I try to discipline myself to use a rowing machine, even if it's for a few minutes. I believe in what I have read about pushing yourself to run when your body is too tired...that can be a setup for injury.

Once in the past I lived five miles from my job, so I was able to get up at 4:30 a.m. and run to work. I used to think that I couldn't run unless I had time to wash my hair after running, and that can be a deterrent for women. My hairdresser advised me to just let out that ponytail after a run and move on to save time. I have actually had people tell me that my hair looks particularly good on days that I ran and never washed it.

Injuries

I have been injured and I often feel little "tweaks" in my body. But I also I think runners can become oversensitive to their bodies. Sometimes it is good to just let it a "tweak" go because 10 or 15 steps—or even half a mile—later, it may be gone anyway. You have to know when to pay attention to your body and when not to.

A few years ago I thought I should get into cross-training and was doing duathlons. I have a good bike, a necessity to compete in duathlons. But I found that I didn't like biking as much as running. Also, I was braking down hills because I didn't feel safe going at full speed. In the transition at a duathlon, I had a mishap and twisted my knee, which resulted in my losing about one and a half years of distance running. I am just coming back to long-distance running from that injury. I used physical therapy, chiropractic treatment, acupuncture, and patience to recover. I did not go to an orthopedist because I knew I did not want surgery. If I cannot run because of an injury, I will do some biking to maintain fitness.

My quads were severely injured running the downhills in my first Boston Marathon. I used acupuncture and chiropractics to heal. I continue to see an acupuncturist regularly to maintain my health and keep my energy channels open. If I sustain a minor injury that concerns me, my acupuncturist can usually employ an appropriate therapy to gently resolve the issue. I also feel it makes sense to utilize chiropractics, since distance running can place unequal strains on the body. I go to a chiropractor once every few weeks to have my body realigned. I've been using these two therapies for about nine years now and have become so committed to them that I don't want to know what my body would feel like without them. I prefer to see medical personnel who involve sports in their own lives, because I think that then they are more sensitive to runners' concerns, and the fact that a runner's goal is *always* to run again.

Current Goals

I just met one of my running goals recently, which was to see if I could still run a marathon at 60. I turned 60 in May and was planning to run the Philadelphia Marathon in November (which I did), but decided to run the Atlantic City Marathon in October first since it was so close to where I live. I won my age group, possibly because I was the only one in it. But, as Michael always kindly reminds me, I beat all the women who didn't show up.

Benefits

I'm a registered nurse, a job with long hours that can be very physically challenging. I manage this work with a lot of energy, which I attribute to running. I don't feel that my energy levels have changed since I was in my 20s, although as I've gotten older, I do find myself tiring in the early evening and needing more sleep.

I try to reserve my running time for myself. I'm much better at it now than I was at first. If I'm concerned about anything, I try to push it out of my consciousness. I read about a lot of runners who think about their life issues or review their "to do" list in their heads as they run. I don't find that that works for me. I want to be in the moment as much as possible. That's how I feel more refreshed after a run.

If I've been sick or unable to run for a week or two, I feel a void and I have to lace up my shoes and get out there, even if it is for a short run.

In the Future

I plan on running as long as my body will let me, and after that I plan to maintain some kind of forward motion! I know I will get slower with time. I love seeing women runners older that I am who continue to run. They are so motivational. I hope to be able to gracefully accept when running 26.2 miles doesn't make sense anymore. When I go online to check the results of races, I usually look up the oldest male and female participants. It's encouraging. I think that all race award ceremonies should start with the oldest age groups.

Postscript: In the year and a half since the interview my son, who was training for his first marathon, has completed not only many marathons but has become an ultra runner. Also, my oldest daughter who had started doing triathlons, now does one a month (in season) and is a member of a women's tri club. It's important to stress that, by example alone, children are prone to mimic your life style.

DIANE MCMANUS
Upper Darby, Pennsylvania

June 2011

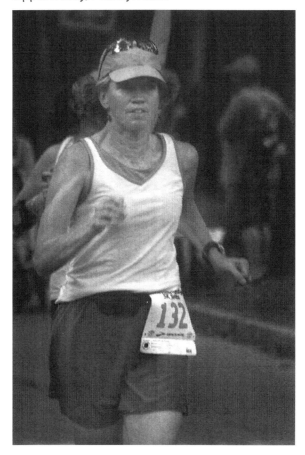

Courtesy of Tony DeSabato

Age: 60

Started running: Age 35

Current training per week: 20–35 miles, varies, depending on race goal

Long run: 8–14 miles, depending on time of year, target race

Best race: Philadelphia Marathon at age 45, 3:54:47

In 2007, after weeks of intensive training, I lined up for a 5.25-mile swim across the Great South Bay from Fire Island to Long Island. This race required all swimmers to have an individual kayak escort. Once we were under way, I relaxed, began to enjoy the experience. By three miles, the water was getting choppier, and I became seasick. As the swim progressed, I felt worse. Still, I finished. My confidence soared: I could hang in through seasickness and finish something that most people had not done. Many have run marathons. Not so many can swim that far across open water.

Early Years and Family

I was born in Boston, Massachusetts, in 1950, the third of (eventually) seven siblings. When I was a tot, my family moved to Pittsburgh, where my father, a pathologist, assumed his new position. We were an active family, although more by way of simply playing outdoors and swimming than in organized sports. My siblings participated in various sports, but I don't remember our being super-competitive. I never married, although I have a longtime close friendship with Neil Weygandt, known for his 45-year-long Boston Marathon streak, among many other running accomplishments.

In 1965, at the age of 15, I lost my father. It was a difficult time—my body and my life both undergoing changes. In 1968, my mother remarried. Since her husband taught at the University of Pennsylvania, my family moved to the Philadelphia area, which has been home ever since. To adjust to the change I would take long walks by myself, or what seemed long to me: four to five miles, much-needed time to be alone, to think things over.

I attended an all-girls' Catholic high school in Pittsburgh. There were a few team sports available—basketball stands out in my memory—and cheerleading. I didn't have the athletic ability to join either activity, but I did enjoy the games as a spectator, and the socializing. After graduating high school in 1969, I attended what is now Franciscan University of Steubenville (in Ohio), formerly the College of Steubenville. As with high school, my college offered few sports—I believe only basketball and club football, both open only to men. Sports weren't my focus, except for swimming during the summer, which I always enjoyed.

After finishing college, I worked at a library, and then returned to school—Temple University—for my master's and doctorate degrees in English. Again, swimming was my sport of choice, a way to relieve stress. Although I had no wish to run, I wondered how people could keep running for a half hour or more at a time, when I would be winded after maybe a hundred yards. Still, I kept up my walking, as a way to get out and experience nature.

I stayed glued to the TV for the 1984 women's Olympic marathon, the first time the event was offered for women. As Joan Benoit widened her lead, flying through the streets of Los Angeles, I was in awe—here was a woman so focused, so fast. When she crossed the finish line as the winner, it was a victory for all women athletes—or aspiring athletes, a defining moment not only for women's sports but for women.

Getting Started

In 1985, I noticed a magazine ad for Outward Bound, an outdoor adventure organization, and sent for a catalog, then signed up for a course. Obviously, I had to get into shape to participate, and among the activities recommended was running. My first attempt was pathetic. Setting out at 6 a.m. to avoid embarrassment, I started running down my street. At first, it was a freeing sensation. The sun was coming up; azaleas were in bloom; the air was cool and fresh. That lasted about two hundred yards. Then my lungs screamed for mercy. I was sure I would die. But something compelled me to try again. People did run, after all, without dying. A friend at Temple University, a runner, invited me to run with her at the Temple gym. Eventually, I was able to run a mile, although my time was slow. Still, my friend encouraged me to try a race. But I had no idea how to go about this and was in no hurry to find out.

I kept up the running, though, and in 1986, after the Outward Bound course, I became more interested in the outdoors, took up hiking, and eventually settled on running. Meanwhile, I took another Outward Bound course in 1988, sailing for women over 30. In this course, we ran daily, and I grew to like it even more. It was time for an honest pair of running shoes. Previously, I had run in an old pair of Sears sneakers labeled as "running" shoes, which wore out. I then bought a $20 pair of Nike shoes from a bargain sneaker store. Finally, I went to a real running store and bought a pair of New Balance® shoes. I had cast my lot with running. In 1988, I ran my first race, a 5K. The appearance of so many lean, athletic-looking people intimidated me. Could I really do this? But I'd already committed myself. My goal: not to finish last. It was challenging due to some steep hills. But I didn't finish last. And despite my vow never to do this again, I grabbed some fliers for future races.

Progression

Slowly, I began to improve, bought books and running magazines, ran more races, and joined a club, the Delco Road Runners. In 1989, I decided to try the Philadelphia Distance Run, a half marathon. I had, after all, run my first 10K race on four hours sleep the morning after a party. If I could run a 10K after a night of more alcohol than usual and sleep deprivation—never mind that I'd run an 11-minute pace—I could run a half marathon. Couldn't I?

Yes, but not easily. Lesson learned from experience: never eat or drink anything unfamiliar right before a big race. My mistake: buying at the expo and drinking some tea-like concoction on race morning that gave me a 13.1-mile-long side stitch. After a running/walking pain-fest, I crossed the finish line in 2:27, and decided I was done with the half-marathon—until I ran a 10K personal best two weeks later. If half marathons could do that for my running, I would do more of them—but certainly not a marathon. Right?

Wrong. With my 40th birthday approaching in 1990, I got one of those "gut feelings"—run a marathon on it. As it turned out, the Columbus Marathon that year was on my birthday. It was a perfect excuse to visit my brother Jack, who lived there, and I was fired up to qualify for Boston. But my training had been made sporadic by injuries. The longest I managed to run was 15 miles. Somehow, though, perhaps thanks to a blessing a priest gave me after mass the eve of the race, I was able to start feeling reasonably good.

Still, at sixteen miles, energy flagging and 10 miles left, I asked myself, "Whose crazy idea of a birthday present was this?" Then I remembered, "Yours, Diane." So I pressed on, wanting more and more for the race to be over. Boston Marathon? No thanks! After crossing the line in 5:07:29, I vowed, "Never again." Sound familiar?

Yet, days later, I thought, "If I can finish, maybe I can do better?" Could I, with the right training, maybe improve enough to qualify for Boston? So I posted a sign in a running store in Philadelphia, advertising for a coach. Several weeks later, I got a call from Russell Floyd, whose marathon personal best was 2:40 and who had coached girls' high-school track. He introduced me to more systematic training: interval workouts, weights, and better-quality stretching. It didn't take long for results to show. I improved from a nine- to an eight-minute/mile pace, and as time went on, even dipped below eight minutes. I made large improvements in my second and third marathons. In the 1991 New York City Marathon, my time dropped to 4:30:09, then in the 1993 Columbus it plummeted to 4:01—not enough to qualify. On pace to finish in under 3:50, I "hit the wall" in the last five miles. My mistake was to run too fast, too soon—I paid for it later.

Then, focused on other distances, I ran my first sub-seven-minute mile at an indoor track meet. In 1994 and 1995, I improved steadily, running my best 5K (22:44 in 1995), and 6:02:07 in the 1500 at the 1995 World Veterans Athletics

Championships in Buffalo, New York (now called the World Masters Athletics Championships).

But I still dreamed of qualifying for Boston. The 100th running of the Boston Marathon was approaching, and so was my 45th birthday, which meant five more minutes added to my qualifying time. I would only need 3:55. I dared to hope again. Armed with Russell's training schedule—including long runs, interval workouts, mile repeats, long tempo runs—I came through the Philadelphia Marathon with a time of 3:54:47. It was by far, and remains, my best marathon, not only by way of time but how I felt.

Boston was an exciting weekend with a family get-together accompanying the race. I felt well prepared. In the race, unfortunately, I developed a hot spot on the bottom of my foot, which grew more irritated as I continued. Further complicating matters, the crowds were immense, with much jostling. For the 100th Boston in 1996, entries were available, not only through qualifying by time, but also through a lottery. Hugs and encouragement from my family at mile eight in Natick renewed my energy. But by twelve miles, my foot hurt enough that I considered dropping out. The other option was to walk the rest of the course, but I didn't want to do that.

Being a spiritual person who believes in the "Communion of Saints," I called on the spirit of George Sheehan, a favorite running writer who had passed away a few years before this race. I said to him, "George, I want to finish. Can you help me?" A block or two later, a man was standing in the middle of the road with a box of Tylenol packets. I grabbed one, thanked the man, thanked George, took the caplets, and within about fifteen minutes, felt much better. By the time I reached Heartbreak Hill, I was again feeling wonderful and passing dozens of people.

Timing chips were used for the first time in the 1996 Boston, slimming my 4:39 clock time to a more shapely 4:22. I'd hoped to do much better, but was still happy to have completed the Grand Dame of marathons.

Injuries, Recoveries, and Swimming

Then I developed a succession of injuries and illnesses, so was sidelined for a few years. I returned to racing in 1999, joining Mike Patterson's Peak Performance group. Mike made up schedules as well as holding speed workouts on Tuesday evenings, and my training improved again. Unfortunately, another foot injury in 2002 stalled further progress.

But this bad fortune led to good. I rediscovered swimming, since I needed to stay in shape. Missing the excitement of competing, I entered a mile open-water swim announced at my Y. A mile at the time took me just under an hour. When I checked the results of the previous year's swim, I noticed that the last-place time was 45 minutes. So I was motivated to improve at least enough to finish before everyone packed up and left. As it turned out, I did the swim in about 47 minutes, with one person finishing behind me.

Not long afterward, I recovered from the injury and again increased my running. Then my mother passed away in May 2004. At around the same time, I lost my job. It then felt like an act of courage to run again, because I was still reeling with grief and shock.

However, I made myself run, knowing that I needed it more than ever. And thanks to a friend who was forming a training team for the 2004 Philadelphia Marathon, I decided that it was time to give the marathon another try. I'd attempted a marathon in 2000, thinking that there was the same magic in turning 50 as there was in turning 40, but had to drop out due to calf pain. To try again, I realized, was an invitation to live again, and so I dedicated the training and the race to my mother. Although far off my best time, the marathon helped reignite my courage. When it was hard going during the race, I felt my mother's spirit and the words "Just run to the next traffic cone," and so, traffic cone by traffic cone, I progressed and finished in 4:57.

In 2005, I returned to swimming. Early in the year, I saw an announcement of a masters team forming at my Y. At first, I thought everyone would be so much faster that I wouldn't fit. But when I called the coach and told him my swimming experience, he encouraged me to join. So for several months, I would arrive at the pool at 6:00 a.m. for practice. During that year, both my swimming and running improved. I tried my first ocean mile—terrified at first of even entering the water, I was relieved to reach calmer water past the breakers and even enjoyed the experience.

I also, again, joined a marathon training group. All went well and I thought I might have a chance at making the 4:15 required to qualify for Boston in my age group (55–59). Unfortunately, I injured my knee about a week before the marathon. With some massage and stretching, I was at least able to finish in 5:01. After that, I stayed away from marathons, concentrating on shorter races.

Meanwhile, I heard of a 5.25-mile swim across the Great South Bay from Fire Island to Long Island—the Maggie Fischer Memorial Great South Bay Cross Bay Swim—and those dangerous words formed: "I wonder if I could do that." To swim across the Great South Bay where I'd taken so many swimming and sailing lessons during family vacations as a youngster seemed like a perfect homecoming. So in 2007, after weeks of training (the swimming equivalent of marathon training for runners), I lined up. Unlike shorter swims, this race required all swimmers to have an individual kayak escort. This was freeing, because I just needed to stay with the kayaker, an expert who had worked with marathon swimmers. Once we were under way, I relaxed, began to enjoy the experience—and made a first-timer mistake: didn't take any water or food. By three miles, the water was getting choppier, and I became seasick. As the swim progressed, I felt worse. Still, I finished much better than I expected, in 3:25:12.

My confidence soared: I could hang in through seasickness and finish something that most people had not done. Many have run marathons. Not so many can swim that far across open water.

Current Goals

Currently, my focus is on running. My goals include breaking two hours in the half marathon, raising my age-graded percent to 70 in at least one race on the Mid-Atlantic USATF Road Grand Prix Series, and placing in my age group in that series. The latter is not easy, because the competition in the 60–64 age group is stiffer than I expected. This, though, is good; it means I have to stay on my toes, keep training, and that is what keeps me healthy. I have to be careful about overdoing and getting injured. As I age, I realize that I need to balance the hard efforts with cross-training...

Benefits

I currently belong to the Greater Philadelphia Track Club, for which I compete on the Grand Prix circuit, and the Bryn Mawr Running Club, which I joined because of interval workouts with the club one evening a week. Through these clubs and through racing, I've made some wonderful, lasting friendships. Both clubs raise the bar and call on me to tap into strengths I thought I didn't have, so I'm happy to be part of them.

In the Future

I hope to continue running and swimming as long as I can, so I admire immensely women still competing in their 70s, 80s, even 90s. When I start wondering if I'm too old to keep up my level of activity, I think of these women and am inspired to continue setting goals.

MARY KESSLER
Wallingford, Pennsylvania

August 23, 2011

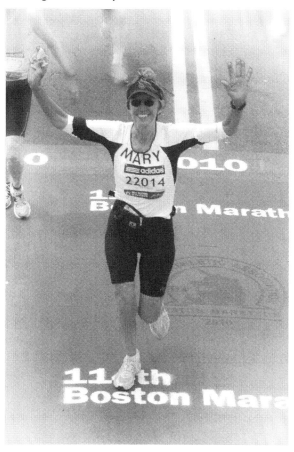

Courtesy of MarathonFoto®

Age: 62

Started running: In my 20s for a few years, then again at age 56

Current training per week: 25–35 miles

Long run: 20 miles

Best race: First Boston Marathon at age 60, 4:24:43

My time (5:20:53) for my first marathon, in Harrisburg, Pennsylvania, in November 2006, was affected by very bad weather. The temperature hovered around freezing with driving rain and sustained 35-mile-per-hour winds! Many runners dropped out. I thought if I could make it through that, I could make it through anything.

Early Years and Family

I was born in rural West Virginia, lived in a house with no indoor plumbing, bathed in a galvanized metal tub on the back porch, kept warm in the winter huddled around a potbelly stove, and attended a one-room schoolhouse. My parents, of German and English descent, were hardworking and dedicated to providing for their five children. Finding employment in rural West Virginia was difficult, so we relocated several times, wherever my parents could find work. We settled in Delaware when I was about eight, and that is where I spent my youth. We moved back to West Virginia right before I entered my senior year of high school.

I didn't participate in sports in high school—at that time, all that was available for young women was basketball. I tried out for the basketball team, but didn't make it. My brothers played football and one sister was a cheerleader. As an adult, my youngest brother became a nationally competitive bodybuilder, but other than that my family wasn't particularly athletic. None of them run.

After graduating high school at the age of seventeen, I moved to Pennsylvania to find work and to create a life for myself. I worked for a large telecommunications company starting at entry level and working my way up to middle management. At the same time I took night classes to earn college credits, and accumulated enough to acquire an associate degree. I had a variety of interesting and demanding positions. As with many businesses, to remain competitive, my employer continued to downsize and expected employees to do more with less. My job was consuming nearly all my time. Nonetheless, it was a great company to work for; I learned a lot, had many wonderful experiences, and was fortunate to be able to retire at the relatively young age of fifty-four.

I've been married twenty-five years with no children. However, my husband and I have lots of nieces and nephews who have kept us busy over the years.

Coming from rural West Virginia, I've always liked being outdoors. I love adventure and have enjoyed hiking, backpacking, camping, and whitewater rafting. I once went on a 30-day cross-country camping trip by myself and, another time, took an Outward Bound sailing course. I've always been interested in health and holistic medicine, and have gone on holistic retreats where

I did some running along with very intensive yoga. I didn't participate in any sports until I started running.

Getting Started

I started running in my twenties because I had friends who ran. One was an avid runner who was selected to participate in a corporate-sponsored relay to carry the 1984 Olympic torch to its final destination in Los Angeles. Running helped me stop smoking too. My friends and I did group runs in the country and speed intervals on the track. I didn't race much—there weren't so many races available in the 1970s. I stopped running in the early 80's when I was working sixty to eighty hours a week and just didn't have time.

One of the things I always wanted to accomplish was to run a marathon, and retirement was my opportunity. So after I retired, I decided I'd better get my knee—which had been injured in an accident twelve years before—checked. At age 54, I had to have ACL reconstruction and meniscus repair, and then had to wait for that to heal before I could start running. I have not had problems with the knee since, a testament to my surgeon and a great physical-therapy team.

A month after surgery I joined a fitness club and began working with a personal trainer, doing what I could within my postoperative restrictions without reinjuring myself. When the time was right in early 2005, at age 56, I started building a running base by jogging on the treadmill because of the soft surface. I read some of Hal Higdon's books and followed his marathon training program for my first marathon. I was so thrilled the first time I was able to break a 10-minute-per-mile pace! My speed and endurance continued to improve.

About a year and a half later I ran my first marathon in 5:20:53, in Harrisburg, Pennsylvania, in November 2006. The temperature hovered around freezing with driving rain and sustained 35-mile-per-hour winds! Many runners dropped out. Friends who came to support me were actually taking off their warm, dry clothing and giving it to the runners who were experiencing hypothermia. I made it—it was a long, long run. Not an ideal initiation to marathoning. But I thought if I could make it through that, I could make it through anything.

Progression

In four years I've gone from a 5:20:53 marathon to 4:16:56, my best, which I ran last fall in Philadelphia. My most memorable marathon is my first Boston, when I ran 4:24:43 at the age of sixty, and qualified to run it again the following year. I've been doing two marathons a year for the last five years using a sixteen-week training program, so thirty-two weeks out of the year I'm in marathon training.

Since my third marathon I've followed the program of the Furman Institute of Running and Scientific Training (FIRST), a group led by scientists and coaches at Furman University in Greenville, South Carolina. They are longtime runners themselves. Their program is documented in a book, *Run Less Run Faster* (Bill Pierce, Scott Murr, and Ray Moss, Rodale, Inc., 2007). Very simply, the program consists of running a specific workout (one speed workout, one tempo run, one long run) three days a week and cross-training two or three other days. The success has been measured meticulously. FIRST hosts a running and learning retreat that I've attended. This involves being tested in a performance laboratory for measures such as Max VO2, body fat, and gait. There is instruction in nutrition, injury prevention and treatment, smart training, and the best strength training for runners. The retreat helped me understand the FIRST philosophy.

My pace and endurance improved with this program, and I feel more fit overall. The program reduces the likelihood of overtraining, burnout, and the risk of injury, as well as being more interesting than simply running five or six days a week. I don't bike outdoors or swim, but I go to spinning classes regularly.

When I ran my first Boston Marathon, I thought I would do it just once. The trip is fairly expensive, but it was so much fun I decided the Sunday night before registration opened to go back again this year. I was one of the lucky people who got in before registration closed after eight hours. Although I requalified (4:21:44), I probably will not go back next year.

I race distances from the 5K on up to the marathon, usually winning my age group in all but the very large races. Since my first marathon in November of 2006, I've run 53 races. I've raced more in the last two years, completing 18 last year. I did the Broad Street 10 Mile Run in Philadelphia once in 1985 when there were just a few thousand people in it, and in 2010 when it was very hot and humid and had 30,000 runners. I'm glad I did it then, but never again. It is much too crowded for me. I prefer the smaller marathons to the very large ones. Steamtown in Scranton, Pennsylvania, is one of my favorites. I've run the Marine Corps Marathon twice; the first time I qualified for Boston. It was lots of fun.

Training Schedule

For every marathon I have an Excel spreadsheet with my three key running workouts, target times/distances, and other exercises. My weekly schedule is:

Running three days, one speed work, one tempo, one long run
Spinning two to three days
Yoga two to three days
Bosu strength one day
Miscellaneous classes I can fit in as needed (Pilates, core strength)

Injuries

When I deviated from FIRST just once, going back to running five days a week, I was injured. Since then I've adhered to the program religiously. Those who are unfamiliar with the program may think running only three days a week is easy, but the three key workouts are quite intense and challenging.

The two injuries I've had since I've resumed running have been to my right leg. This I attribute to inherent weakness in that that leg from my untreated knee injury. When I realize I'm injured, I go to my sports medicine doctor immediately. He diagnoses the problem, prescribes physical therapy if appropriate, and recommends temporary adjustments to my training. He's gotten me through two marathons after suffering injuries just weeks before race time. I belong to a fitness center where I can go for deep-water running, spinning, or an elliptical workout.

I sometimes think my 20-plus-year hiatus from running worked out to my benefit. I know of several people who continued running through their 30s and 40s and are unable to run today to due to injuries and other issues. I believe years of running do not have to lead to debilitating injury; when one can no longer run, it's due to a combination of factors.

Finding Time

I spend two to three, sometimes four hours a day working out, depending on how long and hard I run. Normally, I have the time now that I'm retired. I honestly don't know how people with full-time jobs and families can train for triathlons—or even marathons. The training is so demanding. I am in awe of them!

However, right now my husband and I share responsibility for staying with my mother-in-law in her room in a nursing home. He stays with her three or four nights, usually 20-hour shifts, and I stay with her the other three or four. She's ninety-four years old and quite ill. So we're juggling that right now, along with everything else. I'm finding it very difficult to fit in marathon training. This will be the first year that, because of our family responsibilities, I won't be running two marathons. Right now I'm training for some fall half-marathons.

Current Goals

I hope to continue running marathons, and will when the situation with my mother-in-law resolves itself. I'd like to run Boston again, and I'd like to achieve a PR of 4:15 or less. I'd love to break four hours, but at 62 I believe that a 15-minute improvement is an unrealistic goal. There is a website (www.marathon-guide.com) that lists the marathons with the highest percentage of Boston qualifiers. When I am ready to resume, I'll take that into consideration. I run 5Ks but hate them because I find them painful—I'm running all out and just want the race to be over. Whereas in a marathon, I can just get into a steady rhythm—it's not so painful.

Benefits

The benefits of running are many. I'm fit, maintain a healthy weight, have no health problems, and fortunately don't need to take any medications. What I like most about running is how I feel afterwards. No matter what my troubles may be, or how "down" I am, afterwards I feel calm and peaceful. I have some of my most creative and "deep" thoughts when I'm on long runs. I like the sense of accomplishment. There aren't many 62-year-old women who can run marathons. I see many who have trouble even walking. Although I realize that is not always under their control, many times it is due to years of poor nutrition and lack of exercise. I take personal responsibility for my health and well-being, and my wish is that more women would do the same. It doesn't have to be marathon running, but just do something active for you.

Running is alone time. I am very internally focused. I get lost in my thoughts, so I probably would not be a good running partner, because I don't really like to talk while running. When I'm training, all my runs are timed, so I really can't afford to talk. My only companion during my training runs is my husband. He hates all forms of exercise, but rides his bike with me when I do my long runs in Valley Forge National Park. He's my protector and supporter, and occasionally he tries to coach me—which, needless to say, doesn't work too well.

Diet

My diet is nutritious and well-balanced. I've been a vegetarian for almost 40 years, and am transitioning to a vegan diet. Right now my life is so hectic, and I'm away from home so much, I don't cook as much as usual. It's very difficult to maintain a healthy vegan diet when eating out. For most of my life I have not taken any supplements because I believe that, if you eat a well-balanced diet, they are not necessary. Recently, however, as I have had less control over my diet, I started taking a multivitamin. Also, I've read that as you age, you don't absorb nutrients as readily as when you are younger. I've also heard that processes used to extend the shelf life of foods (so we can have a variety of fresh fruits and vegetables year-round) result in the foods being less nutritious compared to years ago. For these reasons, I'm rethinking my theory about using vitamin supplements. I use Hammer Nutrition's® all-natural products—not only their multivitamin but also Perpetuem®, a blend of soy protein and carbs, for energy without stomach distress during long runs. I also use their gels for shorter runs.

Shoes

The Asics® line of shoes works best for me. I've tried a variety of brands but always come back to Asics®. Before the minimalist shoe movement I tried Nike® Frees, a shoe with minimum support, and was warned by the trainer at my gym to be careful, and not to run in those shoes every day. I support the local running stores rather than buying online or at the large sporting goods stores. I think it is important to have the local stores, with their knowledgeable staff who understand biomechanics and shoe technology. I always buy my shoes at a local store even though they may be a bit more expensive. The staff will let you walk/run in the shoes and make recommendations based on what they see. Some stores have treadmills where they can watch you run and determine what shoe may be best for you.

In the Future

Right now my times are still improving. I'm sure I will plateau and then get slower—that will be a frustrating period for me, because I'm always looking to improve, and finding I'm more competitive than I thought. One day I will have to face reality, but it is not something I want to think about right now. I figure the older I get, the less competition I will have in my age group. There are so many advantages to aging. One thing I know for sure, I won't stop running!

JOY HAMPTON
October 17, 2010

Clarksboro, New Jersey

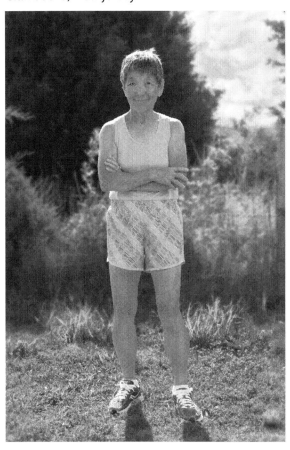

Courtesy of Mike MacKay

Age: 63

Started running: Age 33

Current training per week: 55 miles

Long run: 20 miles when marathon training

Best race: Chicago Marathon at age 51, 3:14

So now I have a 23-year Boston streak. My goal is 25. I will be running my 25th Boston at age 65. I was second in my age group twice in the last four years. (Joy completed her 25th Boston Marathon on April 16, 2012, running 4:07 in temperatures in the mid-80s and placing second in her age group)

Early Years and Family

I am Japanese. I grew up in Japan and all my family is still in Japan. I didn't participate in any organized sports as a child. I was chubby. I did do some winter sports and played a little volleyball. But basically, I didn't do anything athletic until I was 25.

I met my husband, an American, when I was going to college at what is now called Rowan University (New Jersey). My major was accounting but I didn't like it. I took a civil service test and now work for the welfare department as a caseworker. It is a job with a lot of pressure.

Getting Started

I started running because I wanted to stop smoking. I was not a heavy smoker but I enjoyed smoking, especially after dinner. For a while I was running and smoking. One time after the Philadelphia Distance Run, my husband picked me up and I asked for a cigarette. He said, "Nobody smokes here." I said, "I don't care, I want one." I did stop smoking, though it took a couple of years. My husband smoked until about five years ago.

I didn't have any running role models when I started running in the early 1980s. There weren't many older women running. In fact, I was the only person in my neighborhood who ran. I remember watching Joan Benoit win the 1984 Olympic Marathon in Los Angeles. That is when women's running took off. I remember Grete Waitz, who was second in the 1984 Olympics; Ingrid Kristiansen; and Priscilla Welch. A small, red-haired woman named Becky Yankaris, who would now be about 85, ran in Delaware races, but I have not seen her for a few years.

Until my late 40s I ran with no goal. I didn't have a particular training program. I don't do speed work. In 1981 I won my age group in the first race I ran—a 10K. I believe the prize was a medal. I was just happy to finish. I'm always happy to finish. I was surprised that I got an award. I didn't realize I was that fast. I was never really competing against anyone else—just myself.

Progress

It took me a year to run a half marathon: the Philadelphia Distance Run, in 1981. I did a lot of 10Ks. 10Ks were very popular at that time. There was one nearby every weekend. I joined the South Jersey Athletic Club (SJAC) years ago. Somebody tricked me into doing the Grand Prix. I really didn't want to do it, but now they are dependent on me. I very rarely miss a Grand Prix race.

Editor's Note: The Mid-Atlantic Grand Prix is an annual series of 10 races in which local running clubs compete against each other. The scoring is determined by the best age-graded scores of the top runners in each club, and one woman must be included. Joy's high age-graded scores—typically 80 to 85 percent—have helped SJAC win the competition many years.

My first marathon was the Philadelphia Marathon in 1983. That was a hard one. I didn't know anything about marathoning. I was so afraid that I would have to go to the bathroom during the race that I didn't drink any water, and was very dehydrated at the end. I finished in 3:18. I was so overwhelmed that I didn't stay for the awards. My training partner, who was in her 20s at the time, finished in 3:53. In the results book from that race, I found a picture of a good friend running and was able to present him with a copy at his 70th birthday party.

The marathons have become so large. There were not so many people in the races when I started. I can remember when the Philadelphia Distance Run had only 2,000 people. By comparison, in 2010 there were over 15,000 finishers, more than half female. I'm not running the Distance Run anymore. It is too big and too expensive. I've done my 25. In the "old days" we were all sharing the same bathrooms in the YMCA. Now the elite runners receive special treatment.

I do not keep any records of my training or my races. I don't keep my trophies either. Sometimes I throw them away on the ride home from the race. I do know I've run over 60 marathons.

Joan Benoit is admirable in that she keeps competing at a very high level. Many elite runners, like Grete Waitz, stop racing when they slow down in their late 30s. I saw Grete Waitz at a book signing this year and did not recognize her because she has gained weight. Last time I saw Joan Benoit was at the Freihofers Run for Women in 2003. She still looked very thin and fit, and ran a very fast time. She's a very nice person too—had to rush away afterwards to attend an event with her son.

In 1994 I ran the Marine Corps Marathon, and then the New York City Marathon too soon after. I wouldn't do New York again—too many people. Busing to the start in New York and, as in Boston, waiting around for hours at the start, trying to get to the porta potties, is a hassle. I ran the Maui Marathon this year and last. I shouldn't have done it this year—it was too soon after Marine Corps and I hadn't recovered. Old age. Now, if I'm going to run a marathon, I make an eight-week schedule. When I was younger I only needed six weeks.

Editor's Note: Joy won her age group at Maui in 2009 and 2010—in 3:38:31 and 3:52:55 respectively—in very hot weather. In 2010 her time was more than 50 minutes faster than her nearest competitor, and faster than the male 60–64 age-group winner.

Injuries

I did not have any injuries for a long time. Just minor problems here and there. That's because I don't do speed work. Since last year I have had an injury that I think is partly sciatica, partly overuse. A very sore leg. A doctor couldn't find anything wrong with me—just gave me a cortisone shot. I stopped running for a while. Then I went to a chiropractor who is a runner. He thinks he is helping me; I'm not so sure. But overall I've been lucky in avoiding injuries. Just old age now. I do no cross-training, stretching, or lifting weights.

Finding Time

It is hard to find time to train. I work until about 4:30 p.m., come home, change my clothes, and go out about five. I often have to run in the dark. When I get home I cook dinner.

Benefits

One thing I like about running is that you can do it almost anywhere. I also like the mental focus. Just concentrate. You don't think about anything else. You find solitude.

I discovered that another benefit of running is meeting wonderful people. I like seeing them and talking to them after races. I've met so many people from different countries. Otherwise, I'm pretty much a loner. Runners are a different breed. My husband, Bob, is very supportive and proud of me. I can't get him running, though. He has problems with his legs. Bob and I play golf. I love it and have even volunteered in golf events. We have a ping-pong table in the basement. I'm very good at it.

My advice to anyone starting to run is, "Just have fun with it." And join a club. Meet other runners, join in the group runs, and learn from others' experience.

Diet

I don't follow any special diet. I eat whatever I want. I don't consider eating pasta important. I don't digest milk products—including yogurt—well. I haven't used supplements until recently, when my chiropractor suggested I try glucosamine. I haven't seen any benefit yet.

Current Goals

I didn't run Boston until 1988. I wish I had done it in 1984; then I would have run it every year for 26 years. So now I have a 23-year Boston streak. (In April, 2011, Joy completed her 24th consecutive Boston Marathon). My goal is 25. I will be running my 25th Boston at 65. (Joy did that too.) I've always run as a qualifier. I was second in my age group twice in the last four years. Nancy Rollins from Chicago, who is exactly my age, is my nemesis. I beat her in Chicago but she has been beating me the last few years.

I'd like to do the California International Marathon again. It's a nice course—fast downhill.

In the Future

I will run until I can't. My mother lived to 97 and I take after her. So that gives you some idea of my expectations.

SUE BAKER

September 24, 2010

Ocean City, New Jersey

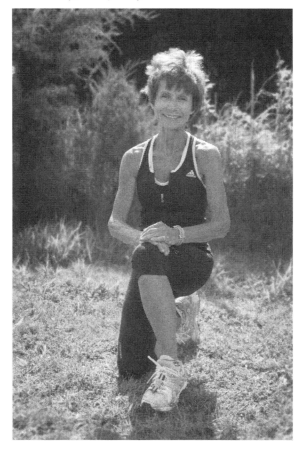

Courtesy of Mike MacKay

Age: 65
Started running: Age 41
Current training per week: 12–15 miles
Long run: Only when training for a long-distance race
Best race: Philadelphia Half Marathon at age 61, 2:17:46, fourth in age group

My husband died very suddenly 16 years after I started running. I read about a Team in Training group here preparing for the San Diego Marathon on June 1. That would have been my 39th wedding anniversary. I thought, "That is how I'll handle June 1. I'll run a marathon in California!!"

Early Years and Family

I was born in Wilmington, Delaware, and grew up on the eastern shore of Maryland. My mother's family came over on the Mayflower. I have two sisters, one younger and one older. My father had a degree in civil engineering, and during the second world war, he built PT boats on the river in Maryland. He loved the area so much that he wanted to stay there. We lived in the country. I rode horses and showed them through high school. I was on the high-school basketball and volleyball teams. Small as I am (five feet and less than 90 pounds), I had a dynamite serve.

I went to Wesley, a junior college in Delaware, for two years. Lynn, my husband-to-be, got a football scholarship to Bowling Green State University in Ohio. I wanted to go there to be with him. My parents wouldn't let me follow a boy to Ohio. So we got married, then moved to Ohio for two years to finish college. We spent our first two summers in Ocean City, New Jersey, my husband's hometown, to earn money for college. We had two boys and a girl, and now have four grandchildren.

My husband had an insurance agency. I became a licensed insurance agent in the early 1980s, and acted as the bookkeeper in our business after our children were in school. The office in Ocean City was across from the elementary school. My youngest son would leave school, cross to the office with a crossing guard, and my workday would end when he came in the door—a perfect arrangement.

Getting Started

I started running in my early forties after I quit smoking. I had been part of a competitive ice-skating team in South Jersey but wanted something more. I'm short and I did not want to gain weight and look "dumpy." Lynn could not run because he had injured his knees playing football, so we bought a StairMaster® to have a good piece of exercise equipment that he could use.

About this time my daughter Kelly was on the cheerleading team at Wake Forest University. Her coach had told the girls that over the summer they had to run a mile every other day to keep in shape. She talked me into running with her because she felt conspicuous running on the boardwalk by herself. This was 1986—when it was not so common to see women runners. When she went back to school I just kept on running.

My goal at the time was just to get that mile in every day. I did no reading about running and didn't consult anyone. I had no role models back then. Later I read a lot of running books and subscribed to *Runner's World*. I follow the Galloway method in marathons and other long races, running ten minutes and walking one minute. It makes a lot of sense to me. George Sheehan's book *Running and Being* (Second Wind II llc, 1998) was wonderful. I read books about nutrition. The more you get into it the more you want to know.

My husband died very suddenly 16 years after I started running—eight years, three months, and one day ago. So that I could receive pension benefits, I ran the business alone for more than five years. There were a lot of stressors, personal and professional. I wondered how I was going to cope.

At the time my husband died, my mileage had gotten up to two or three miles three times a week. I had also been going to the gym three times a week and continued that. I took one day a week off.

I had read marathon stories in *Runner's World* and was intrigued. This was an achievement that no one could take away from you. I read about a Team in Training group here preparing for the San Diego Marathon on June 1. That would have been my 39th wedding anniversary, the first after my husband's death. I thought, "That is how I'll handle June 1. I'll run a marathon in California!!"

I went to the informational meeting at the Ocean City Library. The coach said that he could train anyone to run a marathon. Dan, my youngest son, came with me. I asked the coach if I could do it—I was 57 at the time. He looked at me and said, "Yes, you can. You look fit; you run already." So I signed up. Then Dan said that he would run the marathon with me. Dan was not a runner and neither of us had ever run a race. In training we increased the long run to a new distance every two weeks. I would struggle the first week but be comfortable the second.

Progression

My first race was Broad Street, a 10-miler in Philadelphia, in early May 2003. I went with my Team in Training buddies. By that time we had bonded, exchanged life stories and jokes, etc. We got to the start together, and I had expected that we would run together as we had done in our long training runs. I learned quickly that racing is quite different. Everyone ran their own race. They just took off! They were all faster than me. I was so ticked off, felt abandoned.

But I figured that I had to get down to where my car was parked at the finish. So I ran it. My time was 1:36 and I was 18th out of 46 women in my age group. Very respectable and under my 10 minute/mile goal. I felt fine afterwards.

My next race was the marathon. My time was just a whisker under five hours. That was my goal. I've never done any better. I hadn't made any plans for after that. Running the marathon not only helped me cope with my grief; it also gave people something to talk to me about that was positive. Before, when they asked me how I was doing, I had no answer. Running really helped me cope with my grief after my husband died. It helped my friends too, because it gave them something else to talk about.

I didn't meet any other older runners here for a very long time. I run very, very early, so I don't see many people on the boardwalk. Around Labor Day that year, Dan was visiting and we decided to do the Tim Kerr seven-mile race. We thought, after 26 miles, seven would be a piece of cake. Then we learned that you must train more than two or three miles a day to run that distance. Still, I placed in my age group at Tim Kerr and got my first trophy. The 50s are a very competitive age group and I was at the older end. When I turned 60 I started winning trophies and medals regularly at local races. I've kept them all.

Next, in November, I entered the Trail of Two Cities 5K because it sounded like something interesting to do. The course goes over a long bridge from Ocean City to Somers Point, NJ. I found that the 5Ks were fun.

The year before I turned 60, I told my daughter that I was going to go to Phoenix to do the Rock 'n' Roll Marathon. Kelly had gone to San Diego to watch Dan and me run the marathon. She said she'd really like to run Phoenix and asked if I could train her. I said, "I think I can." She was in her late 30s at the time. I had learned so much from the Team in Training coaches about turning a nonrunner into a running sage. I drew up a training schedule for her. She had moved to Pennsylvania, so I drove to her place every two weeks, and sometimes she came here so we could do our long training runs together. It worked! We ran Phoenix together. She and her 15-year-old son are planning to run the Trail of Two Cities this November. We'll have three generations in that race!

One of the best things about participating in local races was that I saw people in my peer group. When I started running in local races I realized that I was more competitive than I thought. If there is anything I would change it is that I would have started racing much sooner. I thought racing was only for very competitive runners. I didn't realize how much fun it is to be out there with other runners, to meet other runners. Unfortunately, there aren't any running clubs in Ocean City.

I've participated in two other marathons since San Diego and Phoenix: Philadelphia and Steamboat Springs, Colorado. Steamboat Springs was the toughest. There wasn't much oxygen; it started at 8,000 feet and was hilly. I really felt like I was stumbling at the end. Because most people are too sensible to try this race, I ended up with a second place in my age group. Why did I choose that race? We had a family tradition of treating our children to a trip of their choice when they turned 30. Dan was turning 30, and he had his eye on a girl from Colorado whom he had met in Sri Lanka. He suggested that we do Steamboat Springs and socialize with her family. Her father was a runner too. The four of us—Dan, the girl (Bryn, who is now Dan's wife), her father, and I—started together with the understanding that the stronger runners would go ahead when they were ready. Bryn's father was very gallant. He came back and walked with me to the finish.

My most enjoyable race was the 2006 Philadelphia Half Marathon, which is run in November in connection with the Philadelphia Marathon. I was 61 at the time and placed fourth in my age group. I just got into that "zone" and was surprised and disappointed when the race was over.

Training Schedule

I cross-train by going to the gym three times a week for varied one-hour workouts including weight training, step aerobics, and body sculpting. This last year, I've added a 30-minute workout on a stationary bike. I ride a bike, but I am fearful of riding fast outside. I can go very hard on the stationary bikes—great for my quads. I use my StairMaster® every day that I can't get out to run because of weather.

Injuries

Fortunately, I have not had a lot of problems with injuries. About a week after my first marathon I developed plantar fasciitis. I bought a brace and rested. Then after three weeks I decided it was going to hurt whether I ran or not, so I just started running and pushed through it. I've been very careful since to have proper supports in my shoes, and never had plantar fasciitis again.

I have not had any other running injuries. I tore my meniscus once falling on a stair. I did not have to have surgery. Living by myself, I would have had to go into a nursing home for several days if I had surgery, and I didn't want to do that. I went into rehab, and in a cast that made my leg immobile, maintained my aerobic capacity with a hula hoop. After two months I was able to use the StairMaster®. It took four months to get back to running.

Finding Time

I usually don't have any trouble finding time to train. I get up very early and am out and back before the rest of the world wants me for anything. I ran in 14 different races last year; my goal for this year is to do 15. I've only done 11 so far, and since we are past Labor Day it is becoming harder to find races. My priority right now is to sell my current house, and I need to be around to let realtors in. That makes finding the time to race more difficult this year.

Benefits

I've achieved what I first wanted from running, which is keeping my weight down. One unexpected benefit is that my neighbors refer to me as "the little runner." That makes me feel so good. It is so much better than being known as "the little widow." I have a positive identity. And in terms of stress it is cheap therapy. What I like best—and it doesn't happen in training or in most races—is when I get in the zone. Nothing else matters. I'm not old; I'm not young; I'm not married; I'm not a widow. I'm just running. I need that mental break.

I feel much younger than my chronological age. I have women friends my age who act much older. I can't get there yet. I have the same amount of energy as I did 25 years ago, even 50 years ago. As far as day-to-day activities, I feel just the same. I know my running is slower, and there is rarely a race that I don't feel like I'd like to stop in the middle. It's hard. But it is worth it. I know people wonder why I am doing this. In your 60s it is much more significant than when you were younger to come home and feel so good about yourself. I am a runner. The feeling is very satisfying.

I would advise a woman—young or older—who wants to start running to not just run, but become involved in the running culture. You need to train your mind as well as your body. I told my daughter Kelly to subscribe to *Runner's World*. I would advise beginning runners to race as soon as possible. When my husband was alive, my running training and gym workouts did not interfere with our lives because I went out so early. But someone who races has to be at least a little selfish.

In the Future

I plan to give back to the running community. I volunteer in the community in so many ways, and adding running events is something I want to do.

I will run as long as I am able. I don't know that I will continue to compete. Not because of a running problem. Like many runners I have gut trouble. I have to take Imodium two days before I race so as not to embarrass myself. It works, but I'm not sure it is good for me long-term. During a training run you can always cope. I have a trail of porta potties all around the city. When I see doctors, they always do a double-take when they see my resting heart rate. It is so low. But when I explain my gut problem, the response is "Stop running." When you are 65 years old, this is what people are going to tell you.

MILLIE HAMILTON
Redington Beach, Florida

February 18, 2011

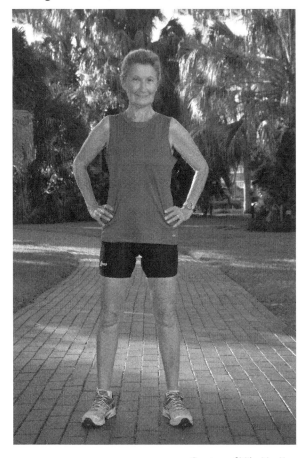

Courtesy of Mike MacKay

Age: 66

Started running: Age 39

Current training per week: 40–50 miles

Long run: 20 miles

Best race: Columbus Marathon at age 62, 4:21:45

I had run the Brandon Marathon in 4:39 at 50. At 62 I qualified for Boston at the Columbus Marathon with a good 4:21:45. I was ecstatic! I believe that the training specific for the marathon, including longer repeats (800s instead of 400s) on the track, made the difference.

Early Years and Family

I was born in Asuncion, Paraguay, and lived there until I was 24. My mother was Italian and my father was a Spaniard from Barcelona. His father was recruited to come to Paraguay following a war in which the country was devastated. Many Paraguayan men had been killed and there was a desperate need for every kind of professional. He was a sculptor, and was brought to Paraguay to build statues to beautify the parks and other public spaces. My Spanish grandmother was a pianist. My Italian grandfather was an accomplished classical musician. Father, while artistic and an accomplished flutist, worked at an auto-supply company.

I did not participate seriously in any sports before I started running. I played a little bit of social tennis and volleyball and swam some, but not competitively. I was not well-coordinated.

In Paraguay my first job was at the U.S. Embassy. One of the teachers at the Embassy encouraged me to apply for a Fulbright Scholarship. I thought it would be fun to go to the United States, so I applied and was successful! I went to the University of Texas first for an orientation, and then to the University of Iowa for graduate work in English.

I was married in Iowa to a man from Fort Madison, Iowa. He was a chemist in an ammunition plant. We lived in Iowa for six years and then moved to St. Petersburg, Florida, for his job. We divorced subsequently. I had worked in a hospital in Iowa and really loved hospital work, so I found a job as secretary to the CEO of St. Petersburg General Hospital and retired as an executive administrative assistant.

I met my second husband, Walter—a physician—at the hospital and we were married in 1986. Walter was a fabulous natural athlete. He played football and ran track in college. He picked up tennis and basketball in his 30s and 40s and played on hospital teams. I got Walter running again.

Getting Started

I started running in July 1983 when I was 39. I remember the date because it was so hot. I was working full-time and my running was sporadic, a few miles three times a week. But sometimes I would not run at all for months. It took me six months to be able to jog a mile without stopping. I was thin—weight has never been a problem—but did not have the natural cardiovascular strength for running. I started at 12 minutes per mile, or slower.

My primary motivation was competition. I had seen a "pack" running in Friday-night beach races in the July and August heat. They looked great. I wanted to improve enough to be part of this pack. There were several women at work who ran Gasparilla, and I figured that racing would motivate me to stick with running. Racing is still my motivator. If I don't have races to train for I slack off, which I don't like to do. My first race was the Gasparilla 5K, which I ran in 1984 in 33 minutes. Pretty slow for a 40-year-old. It was frustrating and embarrassing. I started the first mile feeling really good—much faster than my training pace. I had to walk/jog the last mile feeling very weak. I have a photo that shows I looked awful. I didn't even look the part. Rather than a T-shirt I wore a polo shirt.

Nevertheless, I kept jogging and racing. Once I raced a 5K under 30 minutes I felt better, but I wasn't placing in my age group. The 40s are extremely competitive.

Progression

When I retired in 1990 I went suddenly from running nine miles a week to 30 miles a week. I joined the Sunshine Running Team in Clearwater, a marathon training team. I started doing high mileage, long runs, and speed work on a track with a coach. The Team's goal was running the New York City Marathon. That's when I got injured. I went to higher mileage suddenly—no steady progression. I got a terrible case of plantar fasciitis. For most of that summer I trained in the pool, running using a flotation belt. My long run was three and a half hours in my backyard pool. I made it to New York with the Team and I finished over five hours, like many of the other women Team members who were around my age. This team was more social than high-level performance-oriented. Our aim was to finish; we were called the Marathon Mules—slow and stubborn: you *will* cross the finish line. We had barbeques, runs on the beach followed by breakfast. It was a large group of 50–60 runners of all levels. Being part of that group really laid the foundation for my running career. We went on many fun trips together to races; some of us are still in touch.

After New York my goal was to break five hours in a marathon. The Team always went to New York, but I didn't like that race. I lost about eight minutes at the start—this was before chips. It was crowded and the end was very difficult. So I went with a couple people from the Team to the Twin Cities Marathon. It was a flat course and I ran a 4:57. All my marathons in my 40s and 50s and very early 60s were close to five hours. I stayed with the Sunshine Running Team for 10–12 years, doing a 20-mile long run and a 6 p.m. track workout, which was very difficult during the summer. My training was obviously not optimal because, given my times now, I should have been racing much faster in my 40s and 50s.

I grew tired of the half-hour drive to Clearwater. I had some triathlete friends who invited me go to a nearby track for a 6 a.m. workout with a terrific coach. The track workouts were better and my racing times started decreasing. For three years in a row in my late 50s, I did the Gasparilla "triple challenge." This was a dare to do three races. On Saturday there was the signature 15K followed by a 5K, and then a full marathon the next morning. My goal was to be the oldest woman to complete the series. I ran the 15K and the 5K slowly the first year (age 58) to conserve energy, then had a good massage. The marathon took over five hours. I didn't like that, so the next year I raced the 15K in 1:20:43, my best ever. I walked the 5K because I was "dead," and again had a massage. The next morning I felt pretty good and ran the marathon in 4:49:33. Encouraged, I thought that if I could run that time on very tired legs, with the right training maybe I could run a 4:30 with fresh legs and meet my Boston qualifying time.

I found a very nice specific training schedule in *Runner's World* and a training partner, a Physical Education teacher who paced me. He told me that my 20-milers needed to be faster if I was to reach my goal. He said, "If you want to race a 10-minute pace, you can't train at a 13-minute pace." It worked! I had run the Brandon Marathon in 4:39 at 50. At 62 I qualified for Boston at the Columbus Marathon with a 4:21:45. I was ecstatic! I believe that the training specific for the marathon, including longer repeats (800s instead of 400s) on the track, made the difference.

So my first Boston Marathon as a qualifier was in 2007 at 63. I had run Boston in 2001 as an invited participant—courtesy of a local priest who was a member of the Boston Athletic Association. I loved the course but was embarrassed that I was running without qualifying. On the bus going to the start, people kept asking me, "Where did you qualify?" I had to explain that I couldn't qualify. I knew I would never come back unless I had qualified.

Running as a qualifier was absolutely perfect. I have requalified in every marathon I've run since then, and will be going back this April for the fifth time. Now I only need a 4:45, which is relatively easy. I plan to go back as long as I can. Walter—who has always been extremely supportive of my running—and I love the trip, the race, the whole experience. I am concerned, though, because Boston is raising its standards by lowering the qualifying times.

Normally, I race every second or third weekend. I race all distances from 5Ks to half marathons. I started winning my age group in local races consistently in my late 50s. In my late 50s I was running 25-minute 5Ks consistently, something I could not do in my 40s or early 50s.

Training Schedule

I'm training really hard and long right now. I run five days a week, taking off the day before and the day after my long run. I belong to the West Florida Y in Clearwater, where I run track at 5 a.m. every Tuesday. We do a very long, demanding track workout that is between seven and eight miles. My main regret is that I did not train like this in my 40s and 50s. My times would have been much better. We lose 3 percent aerobic capacity per year in my age range, according to what I read.

I swim regularly. Every Wednesday I go with friends to Fort de Soto to do what we call a mini-tri. We swim, bike, and run. In the winter I swim at a heated pool, but in the summer I join a group on Friday mornings that has open-water swims, and then has breakfast at the house of one of the participants. Swimming may help my running because, they say, it raises your heart rate and lung capacity substantially. I also stretch some after a run when my muscles are warm. I have all the "toys" such as stretch bands and rollers called The Stick®, which are wonderful for massaging your calves especially. I do not do weight training, although I think I should.

Injuries

I have not had many injuries besides the plantar fasciitis I experienced when I increased my weekly mileage dramatically and trained for the New York City Marathon. Someone I knew told me then that I really should cross-train, do some swimming—so I thought, "Why not try a triathlon?" My first tri was in 1991, just a short sprint distance near Orlando. I bought a new bike, but it was a hybrid, not a true racing bike. I wanted to be safe. Walter did a few triathlons with me. He was a very good swimmer. When I turned 60, I decided that I wanted to do a half Ironman. That was a mistake. It was in central Florida and very hot. I wasn't trained for it and I almost didn't finish. I've finished every race I've started. I've never "DNF'd." I've stopped doing tris.

My only other significant injury was to my left ITB band, which is still weak. I went to a physical therapy clinic that was excellent for sports rehabilitation. They got me back in shape using weight machines and an unusual exercise: running through uncooked rice in a kind of hot tub. A physical therapist was with me and pushing me the whole time.

Finding Time

When I first started I would run right after work, before going home, because I found that if I went home first, I had trouble getting back out. I could not master getting up at 4 a.m. to run, and then going to work. I lived near the beach and so I did a lot of beach running.

Diet

In my late 50s I adopted the Paleo diet, also known as the caveman diet, a way of eating that best mimics diets of our hunter-gatherer ancestors—eggs, lean meats, seafood, vegetables (especially roots), fruits, and nuts. I had been eating too much starch and not enough protein. I substituted fruit and vegetable carbs for bread and pasta. I immediately lost 10 pounds, going down from 108 to 98, a better racing weight for someone five feet tall. I adhered to the Paleo diet strictly for several years, through the Columbus Marathon, and I wish could be on it now. I was forced to eat more protein to fill myself up. Roots were an important part, as were all nuts except peanuts.

I drink Gatorade® on my long runs. I hide a Gatorade® in a bush and come back to it. I take only water on my short recovery runs. I take a multivitamin and fish oil daily, and have been told that I should start taking calcium.

Current Goal

Age is really the main barrier to achieving my goals. I am hoping to continue going to Boston until I just "blow up."

Benefits

One obvious benefit of running is weight control, something I did not consider when I started. I also am in much better health than my nonrunning friends. I've never had an MRI or a CAT scan or surgery of any kind. The only medication I take is estrogen replacement. Is it running? Or is it genetics? Who knows? Running has brought me a fantastic social network of wonderful friends. All abilities. All age groups. All encouraging. It's great to be part of the running community.

In the Future

I have volunteered for races when I'm not competing. I might consider getting involved in the organizations: running for the board of directors of the St. Pete Road Runners, for example. I was once asked to be the director of registration for the Turkey Trot, a huge race here of 15,000 participants. It sounded simple, so I agreed. It was basically a full-time job full of problems. Fun but a lot of work.

Most women don't run in their 70s. Many of the superstars here who were doing 3:20 marathons in their 40s aren't running anymore. Not just from running injuries. Many have serious diseases; for instance one extraordinary runner has fibromyalgia, and is in a lot of pain. Why would this happen to someone so well-conditioned?

I would probably be devastated if I couldn't run. My nonrunning days now I fill with gardening, but I know I will be running the next day. I would walk if I couldn't run, or even try competitive swimming. I like competition, not team sports. Swimming is something that we can do well into our 80s.

Postscript

Millie was named to the Florida's Finest team that ran the 2012 Walt Disney Marathon. Made up of 10 top runners in the state, Florida's Finest receive VIP treatment including free entries, free hotel rooms at a Disney resort, free meals, use of a dedicated hospitality suite, a plush tour bus to take them to start, low numbers, and spots in the first corral. In spite of suffering from nagging cold/flu symptoms during her last few weeks of training, Millie ran strong and won her age group in 4:35:42, five minutes faster than her nearest competitor.

FREDDI CARLIP   September 2011
Lewisburg, Pennsylvania

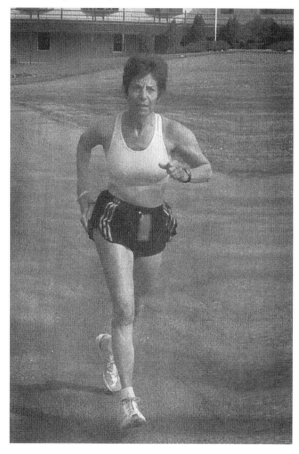

Courtesy of Brent Bacon

Age: 66
Started running: Age 33
Current training per week: 20–25 miles
Long run: 4–5 miles
Best race: Running for Peace 10K in Israel, 2001

I founded the Buffalo Valley Striders at a time when it was unusual for a woman to be president of a running club. I also joined Road Runners' Club of America (RRCA). It was a revelation that I could be accepted in the running community and not get teased, as I was in school. I was on the board of RRCA, the Pennsylvania state representative, the Eastern director, vice president, and then president (2000–2004).

Early Years and Family

The image of a woman I used to know is burned into my mind. She's the foundation upon which my life has been built. She helped me get to the starting line of the run that has become my life. Let's see if I can describe her...

The young woman's life was mapped out by her parents, by the Northeast Philadelphia Jewish community to which she and her family moved from South Philadelphia when she was four or five years old, and, of course by Doris Day and Donna Reed. The only physical activity she ever imagined was giving birth, and perhaps golf or tennis if her social circle demanded it or it helped her husband's career.

She entered college as an Elementary Education major in 1962 at Temple University. The joke on campus was that any college girl studying Elementary Ed was really going after her MRS degree. Her parents thought teaching was the best plan for the girl's future. She really wanted to be a writer.

She had no interest in anything athletic—except her hometown sports teams. She was forever being told she was terrible at sports...and she believed the words she heard. Her classmates laughed when she had to run during gym. She was always chosen last for neighborhood pickup games of any kind. She laughed when the kids laughed, but she hurt inside. She dreaded gym the way most kids dread calculus.

All proceeded according to plan—engaged in her senior year of college, married a month after she graduated, taught school, got pregnant, had first child, second child...Stop!

Here's where life's plan, as arranged by everyone but the young woman involved, had a midcourse correction, thanks to the running boom of the 1970s.

I have been divorced since 1997 and have two children, a son and a daughter—as well as a grandson and a granddaughter—all of them run. My son runs for fitness and my daughter races when she has time.

My daughter and I have gotten through some difficult races together and found love and joy along the way. That's something we can share. The first time my daughter beat me, she wanted to apologize, but I told her, "No! I'm proud of you!"

Getting Started

My love affair with running started in April 1978, when I was 33. As a mom with two small children, I had a lot of stress, and my husband suggested running to help me cope. At first it hurt, but after a while I managed to run a whole mile. At that time, women were not seen on the road. There were no running clothes designed just for women. I wore sneakers. There were no sports bras. I wore my nursing bra, because it was comfortable.

When I entered my first race in October 1978, I bought running shoes—Brooks® Villanova—and men's shorts. The race was the Bull Run Run, a 10K, which I ran with a friend. Our training consisted of running two miles, three times a week. We walked/ran, whatever we could do to keep going, but finished dead last. Even so, we were excited just to finish. We each got a shirt and water. There were no age groups, except under 30 and over 30, and not many women.

Women who ran were a novelty then. There was a lot of sexism. People would say, "You don't want to beat your husband." When I lobbied for equal age-group awards for women, I was called a "women's libber."

Progression

It was after my husband left me that I began to enjoy running for its own sake, by myself. Until then, I always ran either with my husband or a friend. Now I run by myself, for myself.

I've run many races since that first 10K. But perhaps the most memorable was the Running for Peace 10K in Israel, in 2001. There were people of all backgrounds from all over the world. I am Jewish, and this was my ancestral land; I was second in my age group, and I still have the trophy prominently displayed. I got to see relatives who lived in Israel. Someone had to tell me that I placed, because I couldn't read the results, which were in Hebrew.

To stay in shape and be ready for all my races requires that I commit to running. In spite of many other time-consuming responsibilities, I always make sure to get out the door; I get up very early if need be. I also make sure to go to the gym.

While there were few women competing, there were trailblazers. One of my role models was Grete Waitz. She was so composed, made it look so easy. It was a joy to watch her. I also admired Kathrine Switzer and Julie Brown, who ran in the late 1970s and early 1980s, as well as Doris Brown Heritage. They showed what women could do and inspired me early on.

I founded the Buffalo Valley Striders at a time when it was unusual for a woman to be president of a running club. I also joined Road Runners' Club of America (RRCA). It was a revelation that I could be accepted in the running community and not get teased, as I was in school. I was on the board of RRCA, the Pennsylvania state representative, the Eastern director, vice president, and then president (2000–2004). I also served as managing editor of RRCA's 40th-anniversary book.

My commitment to the running community deepened with the years. I am now on the committee for a local race, write a Miss Road Manners column (since 1999), and work with race directors and my township to promote safe running, as well as running and cycling etiquette. I am on my township pedestrian-bicycle committee.

I'm not training for distance now. I run four to five times a week for a total of 20 to 25 miles. The other days I go to the gym to ride a stationary bike or lift weights. As we get older, it's important to mix training. Working with weights helps prevent osteoporosis.

Injuries

We have to make sure we take the time we need to recover from injuries. I've had my share. After my first marathon, in 1983, I jumped up in the air when crossing the finish line and hurt my knee. Then I didn't take enough time to rest. I have also sprained my right ankle badly on runs. As a result, that ankle is more vulnerable to sprains, and I now wear supportive shoes. In the 2002 Philadelphia Distance Run 5K, my leg cramped. I was dehydrated, felt a rip, but kept running and partially tore my soleus (a calf muscle). I was still second in my age group, but needed a long recovery. It took six weeks to heal. Other injuries include a tibial stress fracture. During the recovery, I couldn't run or exercise, just rest. I could do some weights and easy stretches, nothing more. I've had ongoing piriformis problems that I treat with lots of stretching.

One especially galling injury occurred in 2005, when I was running and a storm came up. I passed an orange sign saying MEN WORKING, when suddenly the wind blew it into my shin, causing a deep bone bruise. I was out for three weeks, had to use crutches, and needed physical therapy. Fortunately, aside from these injuries, I've stayed fairly healthy.

Diet

In my diet, I am a big believer in moderation. I eat meat a couple of times a week, pasta, fish, cereal, good bread, fruits and veggies, and yes, I do snack—Chex Mix® is an indulgence. As I get older, I realize there's no reason to not enjoy food. I have a weakness for ice cream, anything chocolate, and I indulge. Still, as we age our metabolism slows down, so we have to be more mindful of what we eat and how much. I am a huge milk drinker—always have been—so I have milk with dinner. I drink wine too. It's got health benefits and is good for the soul.

I eat lots of ethnic food and love to try new things. And good Jewish deli is my comfort food. I have blood-pressure issues, so I stay away from salt as much as I can. I don't add it to food. I love coffee and have it in the morning, and drink tea during the day and in the evening in the cooler months. It's very important to drink lots of water, too. I have water with me most of the time.

My favorite quote is from *Auntie Mame*: "Live, life is a banquet and too many poor suckers are starving to death." This applies to food and to life.

Advice to New Runners

My advice to new runners would be to take it slow. Walk and run at first. Don't rush into a race or get burned out by doing too much too soon. There's no need to run a marathon three months after you start running. Don't give in to pressure. Do what's best for you. Just run and enjoy the experience of hearing your feet hit the ground. Whether you run alone or with someone else is your choice. But get out the door. Running should relieve stress, not induce it. When I run, I create poems, work things out, experience what's out there. For that reason and also for safety, I recommend that you don't wear headphones. Pay attention to what is around you.

Current Goals

Formerly being super-competitive, I now run for enjoyment, my longest races being no more than about five miles. My main goal is just to keep running and enjoying it, although my other commitments can make this a challenge.

I also like to stay active in my community. I'm vice president of the Union County Democratic Committee, and work with a group called Girls on the Run, which helps train young girls, and gives them running partners and other bonding experiences. I help with the Stop the Hate Rally and belong to the Committee to Promote Respect and Equality (CARE). Finally, I volunteer for the Pennsylvania Health Access Network, which provides health care to low-income Pennsylvanians.

More personally, I enjoy writing poetry, watching old movies, getting together for "Girls' Nights Out" with friends, and being with my family. I write social columns for two local daily papers.

And I want to be the role model people were for me. What an example we set for younger women runners. When they see us out there, pounding the pavement, testing ourselves in races and on the track, they quickly learn that running is truly a lifetime activity.

Benefits

You guessed it. That nonathletic Donna Reed wannabe is now an athletic independent woman of—wow—66. She has developed into the person I've become; a person I never dreamed I could be.

Running has given me the opportunity to explore my limits, to test my body, and to push myself. My running roots are planted in the first running boom. They've grown deeper and stronger over the years. Hard to believe I'm now a Super-Senior age-group runner—and since 1981, the owner, publisher, and editor of *Runner's Gazette*, a monthly newsletter for central Pennsylvania and nearby Maryland. I have been involved in running in many ways that have enriched my life, almost from the start.

Women find that their 50s (and beyond) are a transition time. Their bodies are changing, and in many cases, their lives are too. They may be dealing with everything from hot flashes to insomnia, from an empty nest to the death of a parent. At no time in their lives is running as important as it is then.

Our runs give us time to connect with friends or time for some much-needed solitude. Every step we run staves off osteoporosis and lessens the effects of menopause. We can look in the mirror and say to ourselves, *Look at me. I'm strong. I'm fit. I'm ready for anything.* There's no way we'll make ourselves young, but if we stay fit and healthy, we make the aging process that much easier.

In the Future

I sure as hell hope to be running as long as I am able—in 20 years, when I'm 86...and longer. I hope that if I can't run, I will walk. And I will stay involved with running in whatever way I can.

CAROLE L. LELLI
Ocean City, New Jersey

June 24, 2011

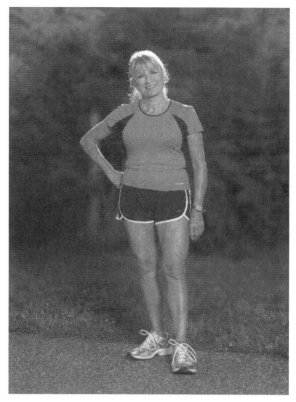

Courtesy of Mike MacKay

Age: 68

Started running: Age 40

Current training per week: 20–25 miles

Long run: 11 miles

Best race: New York City Marathon at age 48, 3:18

My goals when I started running were to replace smoking, maintain my weight, and be fit. I then took it to the extreme. Running has helped me stay young, fit and healthy. And I've made many friends in the running community. It happened naturally. I want to continue running as long as I can—and if I'm not able to run, I'll walk, dance, ride a bike, or go to the gym. I don't plan to ever give up exercise; I'm addicted to it and that is a good thing.

Early Years and Family

An only child, I was born in Vineland, New Jersey, and lived there until I was twenty. I married another Vineland native, an officer in the air force, and moved to an air force base in Texas where two of our three sons were born. Our third son was born in Missouri. We eventually returned to Vineland to be near our families. We divorced and several years later I moved to Ocean City, New Jersey, and have lived there ever since.

Through the years, my dad and mom were my greatest fans. They came to most of my races. Sometimes the whole family came when I ran marathons. My dad was not athletic through sports, but fit because as a nurseryman, he worked outside landscaping and tending to his five acres of nursery stock. My mother was also not athletic, but always encouraged me. I went to a Catholic school where the only sport for girls was intramural basketball. I wasn't very tall, so I did not do well playing basketball.

On my fortieth birthday, in November 1982, I threw out my cigarettes and quit smoking. Although I did not have any health problems, I wanted to watch my three sons grow up and to see what their lives would be like. They were my motivation to quit. It was one of the most difficult days of my life, but I got through those first few months by drinking a lot of water, and eating carrots, celery, and fruit. I worked in a physician's office and could see what happened to smokers as they aged. Smoking led to heart disease, emphysema, and many more health problems, and I had already been smoking for twenty years.

Getting Started

I joined a gym and started taking aerobic classes and lifting weights because I did not want to gain weight. At that time my brother-in-law had just run the Boston Marathon. I was impressed that he looked so fit and could run 26.2 miles. So in April, after I had been working out in the gym for a few months to get into shape, I decided to try running. I ran two miles the first time—checked the distance in my car. I loved running from the beginning. My neighbor, a runner, started giving me old copies of *Runner's World* magazine and they became my "bible." The magazine had articles on nutrition, on how to start running, on how much to do, and on what not to do. I devoured those magazines every month.

Progression

My first race was the Vineland 10K in August of the year I started running, and I ran a 1:10. It made me so sore I didn't run again for two weeks. I learned to pace myself after that and started racing 5Ks, 10Ks, 10-milers, and half marathons as my fitness increased. On the anniversary month of my first year of running, I ran the Philadelphia Independence Marathon in a time of 4:09. I had followed a training schedule I'd found in a book, running the prescribed miles daily.

I started winning my age group soon after I started running. After two years I was winning consistently. I went back to the Vineland 10K, my first race, and placed first overall among females! I have been fortunate to win many plaques and trophies in the 28 years I have been running. I've run 31 marathons to date. Among my favorite races are the Broad Street Run and the Philadelphia Distance Run. My fastest 10-mile time was 1:03 at Broad Street. I won my age group once in the mid-1980s, beating several of my contemporaries, and they were saying, "Who is she?" I was unknown at the time. These women eventually became my "running" friends.

While I was still working in the medical office, I taught aerobics and weightlifting part-time at a local gym. When my boss retired, I decided to open my own gym. Prior to that I had taught a night aerobics class in a nearby church facility. The attendance was good. When I opened my gym the people from the aerobics class came, giving me a ready-made clientele. I hired several instructors. We all completed the courses necessary to be certified in the types of classes we taught, and as personal trainers, as well as learning CPR.

We taught aerobics for two years, then added weights and a few cardiovascular machines so we had a complete fitness facility. I ran the facility for about ten years. I hung my running plaques and awards on the walls to give myself credibility. People began asking me how to start running. So I formed a running class. This was before the days of Team in Training and similar charity training programs that are so popular now. I put an ad in the paper and actually got takers—four guys and three girls. We started out walking a block, running a block. I picked a local 5K and they trained for it and ran it. That was their graduation. Most of those people still run—I see them in different places. We have the "Do you still run?" conversation. Usually I can tell by looking at them whether they are still running.

My sons attended St. Augustine Preparatory High School. When I had my fitness center, I ran with the cross-country students after school, as their coach did not run with them. My two youngest sons ran cross-country and my oldest son wrestled, but ran to lose weight to remain in his weight class. I also worked with the school wrestling team, doing calisthenics and aerobics. The goal was to build up their endurance because they had to be out on the mat for long periods of time.

The report of the President's Council on Physical Fitness and Sports came out during the time I had my fitness center. The Council sponsored a competition among the schools. The headmaster at my sons' school knew I was an athlete and asked me if I could help prepare his students for the competition. We did aerobics, push-ups, sit-ups, pull-ups, and other calisthenics to work on both their strength and endurance. Council representatives came to the school and put the students through their paces as I watched and cheered. They each earned a certificate, making me very proud. That year, at the annual sports banquet, I was presented with a plaque of appreciation. Now, when I see some of those students, they say, "How are you doing, coach?" It is a very pleasant memory.

Now my oldest son runs for recreation. He ran a 3:30 marathon in Philadelphia about five years ago. He does his training when he is traveling, as he has little time when he is home with his family. My middle son also runs recreationally. He does yoga and other exercises with his wife. My youngest son is very athletic. He runs, bikes, and does water and winter sports. They all keep fit and that makes me feel good.

In the 31 marathons that I have run, I've had some memorable experiences. In one of the New York City Marathons, I started right behind Grete Waitz and we were talking before the race, but when the gun went off it looked like she flew off the start line! I've run the Boston Marathon several times including the 100th. With terrific support from the marines, the Marine Corps Marathon was always very moving; you felt the patriotism—especially right after 9/11 when we ran by the burned Pentagon. Chicago is a great town and the marathon there was thrilling.

I joined friends in London and we ran that marathon together. The scenery was great, with the finish on the promenade in front of Buckingham palace. In addition to the costumes, one of the curious parts of that race was the smell of cigarette smoke at the start. Apparently, many Europeans smoke before they start running and then light up again afterward. Amazing!

I've run several California marathons: Los Angeles (very hilly), the first Rock 'n' Roll in San Diego, and Big Sur. I ran Big Sur for the scenery, not for time. It is a very challenging, hilly course. I enjoyed seeing whales playing in the surf and all the colorful field flowers along the way. My son who lives in California always came to watch my marathons there—great support. I've run two Florida marathons: the first Disney Marathon and the West Palm Beach Marathon.

For years my partner—a runner and race timer—and I have been going to the Myrtle Beach Marathon, the Disney Marathon, and the Marine Corps Marathon, to help our friends who own Athletes' Korner Sports Timing Systems (AKSTS). I've actually given the signal to start at some of these big races. That is very exciting!

I've trained on the Atlantic City boardwalk for years, many times with other members of the Boardwalk Runners Club. So it was a given that I would run the 50th Anniversary of the Atlantic City Marathon. I also belonged to the Pineland Striders, another southern New Jersey running club, and trained with many of the members. I did a Grand Prix series competing for South Jersey many times, and was the masters champion one year.

At a point when I was trying to get faster, I did track workouts using a training schedule sent to me by a running friend who agreed to coach me. Friends joined me as I did these track workouts once a week for two years. Several years later, Mike Patterson, a former elite runner who lived in Ocean City at the time, formed a group here that did track workouts one night a week. Although I really never had great speed on the track, the workouts helped me race faster. I have always been more competitive at long than at short distances.

Now I find it difficult to run in the dark and the cold. This past winter I joined our local community center, which has a well-equipped gym. Although we have a treadmill at home that I use, I started running on the gym treadmill and lifting weights. Since I had been having problems with my knees, my doctor suggested that I work out with weight machines to build my quadriceps and hamstrings to help support my knees. I did this for a few months, and plan to start again in the fall when I have more time.

I have kept a daily log since my second year of running. It's fascinating to me to go back and see the miles I was running and how I trained for races in the past. I trained and raced very hard.

Injuries

I broke my foot a few years ago—not a running injury—and was in a boot for six weeks. I lost a lot of speed then and never gained it back. I have trained for, and run, several marathons since, but not with the same training intensity or race times as before.

I also have a knee injury that has become chronic. I was treated with a series of five Supartz® injections (hyaluronic acid), which are used to replace the synovial fluid in my knee joint. I think they helped, but I'm also putting less pressure on my knee by not running the miles I did in the past.

Finding Time

When I started, I ran in the dark early in the morning and in the evening, not thinking much about safety. I had kids at home, so I had to run before they went to school and after dinner, when they were settled doing their homework. I trained for my first two marathons like that. Later, I met another woman who ran and we began running together at 6 a.m. daily. We are still good friends today and get together occasionally to run.

I worked during the week and raced on weekends when my kids didn't have activities that kept me occupied. Sometimes my family came to the races; other times I went with friends. Most of the time I would just run a race and go home.

Diet

My diet is fairly good. I eat chicken, very little red meat, a lot of fish, vegetables, bananas, and other fruit. Of course, I can kill a bag of potato chips as well as the next person. We eat some pasta, mostly wheat or multigrain, and have cut back on carbohydrates. I don't eat ice cream, but I do enjoy cookies. For supplements I take a multivitamin, fish oil, glucosamine, and calcium. Before a run, I might take a GU, drink some Powerade® or eat something relatively new, Clif Shot Bloks®. I was surprised at how much of a boost they give me.

Benefits

My goals when I started running were to replace smoking, maintain my weight, and be fit. I then took it to the extreme. Running has helped me stay young, fit and healthy. And I've made many friends in the running community. It happened naturally.

This year, for the third time, I entered the Ms. New Jersey Senior America Pageant, which was held in June in an Atlantic City casino. The pageant, for women over 60, is similar to the Miss America pageant but without the swimsuit competition. I finished third in the 40th annual pageant in June 2011. For the talent portion I worked with a dance teacher to develop a routine that involved movement over the large stage. I treated the training like marathon training—same principle. One of the most rewarding aspects of the competition is that, after competing, we volunteer our time to go in groups to nursing homes, senior centers, 50-plus communities, etc., to entertain the residents. My work as a realtor in Ocean City, New Jersey, doing sales and rentals, allows me the flexibility to do this. I enjoy my job, but I also want to continue my work with the pageant.

I encourage people to start running at any age. Get a checkup first and start slowly. Buy a good pair of running shoes so you won't have foot and shin problems—don't go out in your Keds®. Most important, build up slowly (run, walk, run, walk); running can be beneficial at any age. And if you can't run, walk. You'll be able to eat more of your favorite foods, and feel better.

In the Future

I want to continue running as long as I can, and if I'm not able to run, I'll walk, dance, ride a bike, or go to the gym. I don't plan to ever give up exercise; I'm addicted to it and that is a good thing.

SUE LEVY

October 13, 2010

Philadelphia, Pennsylvania

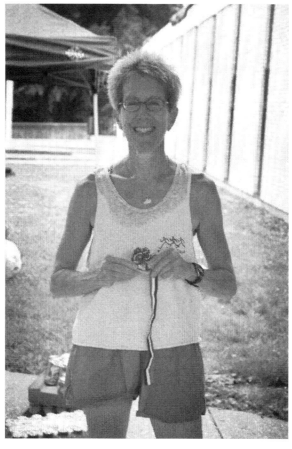

Age: 70
Started running: Age 45
Current training per week: 12 miles
Long run: None
Best race: Anti-Graffiti Run (5K), Philadelphia, at age 48, 23:33

I placed in my age group early on. In my best year, 2003, I ran in 143 races and placed in my age group 133 times. As of the end of 2009 I had participated in 2,310 races and placed in 2,030; 280 of the races did not have age-group awards.

Early Years and Family

I grew up in Huntington, Long Island, with a brother five years younger. I never participated in sports as a child, or in high school and college, or later until I started running. I was not well-coordinated and disliked sports. I did enjoy walking, not for exercise, but instead of taking public transportation.

I was a teacher specializing in early childhood education. I taught both gifted children and mentally disabled children, then joined the Early Childhood Center at Drexel University working with three-year-olds. Subsequently, I became director of the Center and stayed there until I retired 22 years ago.

Getting Started

I've been married twice and have been a widow now for two and a half years and five days. My second husband, Marv, was a runner and regularly raced competitively. He encouraged me to start running. Then, one time when we were on a cruise, I went to the fitness center and started walking on a treadmill while Marv was running. I found I liked it. When we got home we bought a treadmill. Marv wanted me to enter a race with him, and I thought that anyone who raced was slightly nuts. But I did, and I came in last. For that effort Marv gave me a huge trophy that he had made, which said, "First Race," and had other pertinent information on it. I was hooked. I thought that if I can get a big trophy like this, I'll go to races.

Progression

My times improved from 31:50 at that first 5K race in July of 1986 to 24:12 in a 5K in 1987. I know that because I keep a log of all my races and training, noting date, time, and mileage. My husband, who was considerably older than I am, continued to be my primary motivator and role model. He was in great physical shape and always thin. Running and racing was something we could share. The camaraderie and winning trophies were fun, and we enjoyed the food served after the races while we were waiting for the awards ceremonies. I liked the feeling of having done something physical.

I placed in my age group early on. In my best year, 2003, I ran in 143 races and placed in my age group 133 times. As of the end of 2009 I had participated in 2,310 races and placed in 2,030; 280 of the races did not have age-group awards. In addition to a log with distance and time, I keep a folder by year containing the bib, directions to the race, and application. On the bib I write information such as the time, place, food, age groups, who my competition was, and terrain. I attach the directions to the race because I'm directionally challenged. If I do the same race another year, I just pull out the directions.

Training Schedule

In retrospect, I would not have been so hard on myself. I would not try to run five miles before breakfast every day—thought that my world would collapse if I didn't. I would have listened to doctors more. I would have not been so anxious to get back so quickly after injury. And I would not have been such a poor sport.

Now I cross-train three times a week: Monday, Wednesday, and Friday. To develop upper-body strength and to give my legs a rest from pounding, I go to the gym to use the weight machines, stationary bike, and elliptical machine. Tuesday and Thursday I do three-mile training runs, and Saturday and Sunday I participate in 5K races. I have run one 10-mile race and have done two Loop Races (8.4 miles on a course near where I live). I prefer to train alone so that I can go at my own pace.

Injuries

Over the years my running times have slowed. I have been injured many times: broken metatarsal in each foot, stress fracture of the femur, torn gastric muscle, and broken knee. When I was in my 60s I started to get injuries more often. I was a very poor sport when injured. I didn't want to go out to a race, hear about a race, or talk to runners. Not a happy camper. Now that I'm older I take it in stride and just go out and do the best I can.

Surprisingly, I needed open-heart surgery in July of 2008. Knocked my running socks off, as I eat a fairly healthy diet, exercise regularly, and am thin. Mitral valve repair. Cause: genetics. I was back to walking six weeks later!!

Diet

My diet is both good and bad. I eat tofu, yogurt, salmon, fish, chicken, and lots of vegetables and fruit. I eat red meat only a few times a year. After dinner I have cookies, candy, or ice cream. On vacation I'll drink champagne, and eat more meat and rich deserts. I don't drink at home. I take supplements:

multivitamins, vitamin D, calcium, lutein for eye health, and fish oil. I don't use sports drinks.

Current goals

My current goal is to just get out there and run on weekends. I do it now more to socialize than to race. I like being around the people, and especially like the admiration of younger women runners who find it amazing that a woman almost 70 can not only stand up, but run. In the past I treated running like a job. I felt that once I got it out of the way I could do whatever I wanted. Now it is more fun.

At this point in my life I love to travel. I don't run when I travel. When Marv and I traveled we would be sure to book the travel so as not to miss races that we wanted to do. I don't bother with that now, but once I've booked I'll go online to see if there are any races I might do near where I'll be.

Benefits

I've never treated running as a means of losing weight because I think that with the short distances I run, there is not much impact. But running has provided me with a toned body and one that recovers faster than average because of the conditioning. The social part of running was very important to us. We met many nice people who became our friends. Runners are great people. They are healthy, in tune with their bodies. You can have running friends of all ages, male and female. No one hits on anyone.

I belong to some running clubs to support them with a contribution and to receive their newsletters. (Although now you can get all the race information online.)

I'd advise any beginning runner to start slowly—don't go out too fast and don't run too much. Don't be too hard on yourself. Look at the scenery and listen to your body. Meet new people. Enjoy the experience and watch out for cracks in the sidewalk.

In the Future

I expect to run as long as my legs and God let me. I've coped with, and expect to continue coping with, the changes as I age by going with the flow and staying positive and realistic. I try to have a more relaxed frame of mind. If my doctor told me that I couldn't run again, I would go out and walk. I have that to fall back on. However, I try to choose doctors who are runners so they won't tell me not to run.

July, 2011

SANDRA FOLZER
Glenside, Pennsylvania

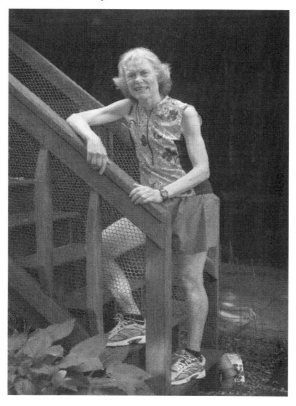

Courtesy of Mike MacKay

Age: 72
Started running: Age 37
Current training per week: About 25 miles
Long run: 10–12 miles
Best race: JFK 50-miler at age 40, 9:01, second woman overall

I'm a 17-year breast cancer survivor, with a double mastectomy. When I run now I feel such support from other runners. When I did Race for the Cure in 1995 while finishing chemo and bald, two of my daughters printed T-shirts for me and some running friends as a surprise. They had angels on them and "For Sandy." When I did that 5K, these runners with their angel shirts surrounded me as I ran. I can cry just thinking of it. It was so lovely. One friend told me later he thought we'd be going slowly, but he had to push to stay with me.

Early Years and Family

I was born in Evanston, Illinois, outside Chicago, the younger of two daughters, and grew up in Evanston and Northfield, another suburb, until I went to college. Both my parents were artists. In high school, I participated in after-school soccer. There was no track. While attending Carleton College in Minnesota, I took archery and horseback riding for gym. In addition to organized or school sports, I played tennis—and in Illinois, everyone went ice skating in winter.

I'm now divorced and living with John Dulik, my partner of 20-plus years, in a house we own together. I have three children and two grandchildren. My daughter Amma was born in Africa, lives in Chestnut Hill, and has two daughters: Anni (age 15), and Marley (age 11). Laura lives in Brooklyn and is happily married, and Victoria lives in Brazil with her Brazilian husband.

I am retired after 30 years as a full professor in behavioral health at Community College of Philadelphia. I was a licensed psychologist. Family is very important to me: I treasure any time with my granddaughters and enjoy traveling with John or my girls. We'll go back to Brazil again probably in 2012 to visit Victoria. I have four cats, which someone dropped off at our house last summer.

Getting Started

My ex-husband was a runner, and I first began running in about 1975. My marriage was not going well, and I wanted to build confidence. At first, I ran around the block and thought that was tough. Fortunately, I soon realized that once I warmed up, it was much easier. About a year later, I ran my first race, the Philadelphia Marathon. Someone had told me I could do the marathon if I could run around East and West River Drive twice (16.8 miles), and so I did. That was my preparation. I ran a 3:45 and came in fifth woman overall.

There weren't many women running when I started, and I didn't know other women runners. Now, I would say Joan Benoit Samuelson is a role model.

She is still running well in her 50s. My advice to women just starting to run: Find friends who can join you, or join a group. Find a regular time to run; make it a routine. Enjoy it. If at first it seems difficult, try a little longer. Running gets easier after you warm up. So many times I have started thinking I had no energy, then felt better, then good.

Progression

I enjoy the sensation of running. I love the camaraderie of running with friends. I run at 6:45 a.m. with a few people who meet at Valley Green, a scenic spot in Philadelphia's Wissahickon Valley Park. We run on a trail deep in the woods that follows the Wissahickon Creek. On Saturdays I run with the Shawmont running group in the Wissahickon. I do my long run with them. During the summer, when I'm living upstate, I run alone or with my partner, who usually runs about half the distance I do. There are lots of hills in Tioga County where we stay. I do a bunch of races there. We try to bike in the summer too.

Nowadays I mostly run 5Ks because that's what is available.

Editor's Note: Sandra won her 70–74 age group in the 10-mile 2011 Broad Street Run, with a chip time of 1:26:39. Based on the WMA age-grading table, this is equivalent to a 56:40 for an open runner. At the age of 47, in 1986, she ran Broad Street in 1:05:09. She has delivered many other impressive performances, including a 38:41 10K (1986), a 19:17 5K (1986), and even well into her 60s was racing a sub-eight-minute pace.

To save my legs, I don't run marathons anymore. In the past, I have done a few marathons and a few ultra-marathons including, in 1980, the 62-mile race between Philadelphia and Atlantic City in 10 hours, 15 minutes. I was first woman. In 1979, I ran the JFK 50-miler in nine hours, one minute. I went because a friend was doing it. At the start there were a bunch of Marines who clearly looked down on me, a woman. They were sure they would blow me away. The course is partly on the Appalachian Trail, so it is demanding. Well, I passed them with gusto and finished at least an hour before they did. Never underestimate a 40-year-old woman! I was 89th out of 405 finishers and second woman.

Besides leading to racing successes, running has made travel more adventurous. When I was in Kenya with a friend and wanted to run, a Masai warrior guarded me from lions with a spear while I ran around a field. Sounds surreal and it was. When I was in Indonesia last January, I found it difficult running in the city. Being in a mostly Muslim country, I also didn't want to offend. Then, I learned that Muslim women would run in covering and only on Sunday. In Bali, which is Hindu, I ran a two-mile loop, passing nine Hindu temples, as well as rice fields. When I was in Barcelona in the 1980s with my daughters, I would run at the break of dawn, since I never saw others running. I ran in long pants in summer, trying to be culturally correct. I found a small park that I would run around. On the way home, I stopped at a bakery to bring treats back to my daughters. The place we stayed in had only cold water, so I had a nice cold shower to greet me after the run. I thought I'd get used to it but never did. In Brazil, where one of my daughters lives, we ran along the beach in Niteroi. It was gorgeous.

Injuries

I have been lucky as far as injuries go, but have had a few. I fell through my barn roof once and couldn't run for the summer. I broke my foot a couple of summers ago from wearing shoes with a metal rod and going fast downhill. Otherwise, I have had only minor stuff that, when I just rested a week or two, was fine. With the broken foot, I swam, and while recuperating, also did an upside-down pedaling exercise to keep in shape (I made it up). I believe I stay injury-free because I usually run four days a week and give my body a rest three days.

Training Schedule

Although I'm retired, I'm still busy, but during the fall and spring when I run with others, I have a good training schedule: I run hills (7 miles up and down) Mondays, do intervals on Tuesdays, off Wednesdays, 5–7 miles on Thursdays, off Fridays and Sundays, and run long on Saturdays (10–12 miles).

Shoes

I wear orthotics. I may have gotten them 25 or more years ago because of an injury. I've been wearing the same orthotics since then. My podiatrist says they are still fine.

Current Goals

My current goals are to stay healthy and uninjured. I would also like to do a 24-minute 5K again, but age is a barrier. I work harder and harder and still get slower.

I have many interests besides running. I write letters to editors about political and environmental issues, as well as a monthly article on the environment for the Weavers Way Co-op paper, and I am chair of their Environment Committee. I am very active protesting gas drilling in Pennsylvania, since the

Marcellus Shale is near my property in Tioga County. I hate to see the pollution and destruction caused by the drilling.

I'm in a book club, write short stories, and have a nonfiction book I'd like to publish. I'm also in two women's groups and have season tickets to the Philadelphia Orchestra, the Arden Theater, the Walnut Theater (where I take my granddaughters), and Stagecrafters Theater..

I also enjoy gardening and cooking. I have two gardens, one in the Philadelphia area and one upstate. I make all my bread, as well as yogurt and granola.

Benefits

I'm a 17-year breast cancer survivor, with a double mastectomy. I think running has helped me recover. I'm healthier than any of my friends. But those friends have been a significant part of my recovery as well.

I feel such support from other runners. When I did my Race for the Cure in 1995 while finishing chemo and bald, two of my daughters printed T-shirts for me and some running friends as a surprise. They had angels on them and "For Sandy." When I did that 5K, these runners with their angel shirts surrounded me as I ran. I can cry just thinking of it. It was so lovely. One friend told me later he thought we'd be going slowly, but he had to push to stay with me.

Since then, I've done the Race for the Cure every year with my daughter Laura. It's our tradition. We came in first among survivors for ten years. Now we have been second for the last five years. Not bad at 71! (My 72nd birthday was shortly after the 2011 race.) I so enjoy the folks I run with. They have become good friends.

This incident is just one of many that make running worth it to me, and shows how important the camaraderie of runners is to the healing process. When I run now, as in the past, I feel such support from other runners. To give back to the running community, I pick up trash when I run. I was on the Board of the Philadelphia Distance Run for many years and have helped at the Philadelphia Marathon.

In general, I enjoy life and have lots of energy.

In the Future

I hope to run as long as my body lets me, even at 92 in 20 years.

GLORIA JENKINS
Westampton, New Jersey

Fall 2011

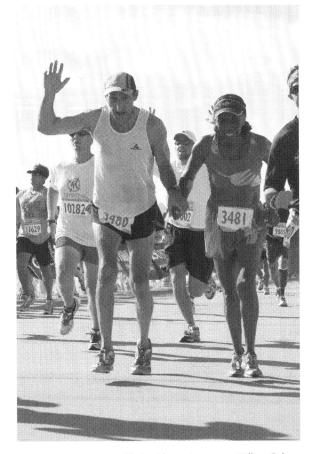

Gloria with running partner William Palese

Courtesy of Marathon-Photos

Age: 73

Started running: Age 42

Current training per week: Approximately 25 miles

Long run: 6–8 miles (as many as 30 miles when younger)

Best race: Marine Corps Marathon, at age 44, 3:09:05

When I was younger, I ran five to ten miles a day, sometimes five miles in the morning before work and ten miles after work with a running partner. Once, I ran from Willingboro (New Jersey) to Bordentown, about 28 miles away. It was the hottest day of the year, and I had only a quarter in my pocket!

Early Years and Family

I was born in Cleveland, Ohio, on November 5, 1937. I went to East Technical High School, was awarded a four-year academic scholarship to West Virginia State, and graduated with honors in elementary education. I was the only one of eight siblings who attended college. I did not have an interest in sports in high school, as I worked to help my mother support the family.

Both my husband and I have master's degrees. My husband, Samuel, retired from the army as a lieutenant colonel. We have been married over 50 years and have three children. All have college degrees. My son, Samuel Jenkins III, graduated from Temple University where he had a five-year football scholarship; my daughters, Saline and Glenna, both have advanced degrees.

I retired in June of 2002. At that time, I was a Learning Disability Consultant with the Child Study Team in Moorestown Township, New Jersey. I have also served as assistant principal in Pemberton, New Jersey, as director of the Child Study Team in Pemberton, and as a teacher (kindergarten through high school), for a total of 37.5 years of public service.

Getting Started

I started running in my early 40s. It was not easy at first. I remember jogging around the block from my house in Westampton, New Jersey, coming into the house, and almost passing out on the dining-room floor. But I got up the next day and tried again...and again. My first real run was at Mill Creek Park in Willingboro, New Jersey (the home of Olympic Champion Carl Lewis). A man from the Mill Creek Runners, a local club, asked me if I could run a 1.75 mile loop in a 10-minute pace, but I misunderstood him. I thought he was asking if I could run the whole loop in 10 minutes, so I tried to do that and succeeded, although it was very hard. The man was impressed, and encouraged me to race.

A little later, I read a newspaper article about a 60-year-old runner who had recovered from a stroke—he learned first to walk around his bed, then the room, and finally outside. He ended up running a marathon. (His recovery took eight years.) I was so excited and inspired by this that I ran all the way from the park, six miles away!

Progression

Eventually, I joined the Mill Creek Runners' team, and in my first four-mile race, I placed second, even though I had on old tennis shoes. Since then, I have raced many times. I peaked in my fifties. At one point, I was ranked 12th master runner in the country.

Racing highlights are the Honolulu Marathon in 1983, 3:24:20 at age 46, where I placed 33rd female overall and 4th in the 40–49 age group; the L'eggs™ Mini Marathon (10K) in 1985, 41:02; and a 6.32 minutes-per-mile pace in Brian's Run (10K) in 1978 when I was 41. I've run eleven marathons, including the 1981 Philadelphia Independence Marathon in 1981 (3:38:31); the 1982 Boston Marathon when I was 43, finishing third in my age group; and seven Marine Corps Marathons in the 1980s with a best time of 3:09:05, also in 1982. I won local races outright (first female) when I was in my 40s.

I had an unusual experience in Boston. At that time, policemen on horses rode along the route to monitor it. When I was about four miles from the finish line, the backside of a horse knocked me over towards the side of the road. A runner caught me. It woke me up! Got me back into the action and helped me finish the race!

Now I belong to the North Jersey Running Club. They are distance runners. We usually run about 10 miles on a hilly trail. I'm also a member of the New Jersey Road Runners' Club and South Jersey AC, and was a member of the Pineland Striders for a while. Often I run with a partner, William Palese. I've raced all distances: 10K, 5K, 4-milers, half marathons, and marathons. I used to race every week. Now it's maybe six to eight races a year. The half marathon in Virginia Beach is the longest I've run in the past eight years, and my favorite race. I've been first or second in my age group in the past five years.

> **Editor's Note:** *Gloria's Virginia Beach Half Marathon times:*
> *2010: 2:19:33, 1st Age Group 70–74*
> *2009: 2:13:59, 1st Age Group 70–74, age-graded 81.1 percent*
> *2008: 2:10:03, 1st Age Group 70–74, age-graded 79 percent*
> *2007: 2:03:36, 2nd Age Group 65–69, age-graded 81.7 percent*
> *2006: 2:15:33, 2nd Age Group 65–69*

Once my marathon time hit four and a half hours I said, "That's it; I'm not doing that anymore."

I placed first in 1987 (1:11) and second in my age group in 2008 and 2009 in one of Philadelphia's premier distance races, the Broad Street Run (10 miles), with age-graded scores over 80 percent. In the 25-plus races I've run in the last five years, I've nearly always been in the top three in my age group, and I was first in eighteen. There are not many women in my age group now, as most have dropped out. In spite of my times being slower as I age, my age-graded scores have been consistently near 80 percent. I feel good about that.

Besides running, I have for the past eight years presented Black History programs for seniors, schoolchildren (storytelling), and other interested groups at no charge. I love flowers and gardening, so I do all the landscaping for my house. Some years back, I participated in three Outward Bound adventures. I climbed over rocks, rappelled down cliffs, spent time in the wilderness surviving on my own, and loved it.

Training Schedule

When I was younger, I ran five to ten miles a day, sometimes five miles in the morning before work and ten miles after work with a running partner. Once, I ran from Willingboro (New Jersey) to Bordentown, about 28 miles away. It was the hottest day of the year, and I had only a quarter in my pocket!

It's hard to find time to train now, and I have forgone races, because my husband is ill and needs considerable care. The kind of training that I used to do takes a lot of time.

Injuries

I have some knee problems, but I'm still out there pushing along the way (no six-minute miles; instead, nine- to nine-and-a-half-minute miles). I have sciatica that causes numbness in one leg, so I do more gym work (free weights) now. My doctor advised me to do dead lifts.

Thankfully, my upper body is very strong; it's something to fall back on when my legs are failing me. You are more prone to injury as you get older, and it takes longer to heal. I believe that injuries are one reason runners drop out. Another reason is simple: Running is hard.

Diet

I eat whatever I want. I can do that because I'm so active. I tend to eat small amounts many times during the day. I don't eat a lot of fried foods. I should eat more fruits and vegetables. My doctor prescribed calcium, fish oil, and other supplements.

Benefits

Running takes the place of many pills. It helps to relieve stress, keeps your weight down, and keeps you looking younger than you really are. (Vanity is my name.) (Smile)

My advice to new runners: Learn to run alone! Group activity is great, but when you are out there on the road, it's up to *you* to make it! Stay strong! But start out slowly and work your way up. People shouldn't race every time they run. Watch what you eat. Enjoy food but in moderation, and take vitamins. Dress properly to stay warm in cold weather. Spend money on your shoes and you save in the long run. Women in particular should do upper-body work and find a man to run with for building speed.

Current Goals

My goal now is to keep running for as long as I can. I would love to run one more marathon before I stop. My friend Lorraine is 80-plus and she's still on the road (over 30 marathons).

I enjoy writing and have written four short-story books, two of which are published: *Storm, the Peace Maker* and *The Surprise Basket*. Besides these, I also wrote two *Be Careful What You Wish For* books, which I want to publish.

RITA ALLES
Hamilton, New Jersey

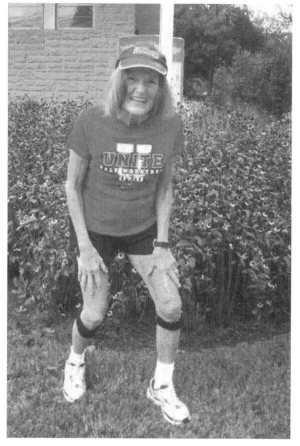

Age: 74
Started running: Age 39
Current training per week: 10–12 miles (limited by injury), plus spinning two days
Long run: 5 miles now, longer before injury and when training for half marathon
Best race: My first marathon, the Avon International Marathon, 1978, 4:01:58

When I was ready to run my first marathon, I was talked into doing the Avon International Marathon that was being held in March 1978 in Atlanta. My time was 4:01:58. In September I went home to Chicago to run a marathon there. Then New York in October; Jersey Shore in December; Miami in January 1979; the Prevention Marathon in Bethlehem, Pennsylvania, in March; and the Penn Relays in Philadelphia in April. That was six marathons in seven months!

Early Years and Family

I was born in Chicago, in the "Back of the Yards Neighborhood," the meatpacking district of Chicago. For a long time I didn't tell people where I had lived before moving to New Jersey in 1966, a couple of weeks after I had my sixth child. Would only say "Chicago." I was born at home on April 21, 1937.

Regarding ethnicity, my last name, Alles, means "all" in German. My father's parents were Czech and Bohemian. My mother's parents were from Poland. I am the second of six children. Two of my younger sisters have run and participated in some races. I did not participate in sports in high school or college, although I walked a lot as a child—we didn't have a car and walked everywhere.

In 1976, I received my Bachelor of Arts Degree from Rutgers, New Brunswick after going part-time for a long time. (That was my first marathon.) The year I graduated, my oldest child graduated from high school. I then started working for the State of New Jersey in Human Services, with clients classified as mentally ill, and later with clients who were developmentally disabled. The job was rewarding, but frustrating sometimes. I retired in 2002 because there was a "buyout" and I had turned 65.

I have been married to fellow runner Dick Hueber for 17 years. We met on the running scene and dated beginning June 3, 1993, and then just happened to get married on June 3, 1994. Both Dick and I were married before. He has three children and six grandchildren. I have six children and twelve grandchildren. We go to watch a lot of our grandchildren's activities.

Getting Started

I played some tennis in the early 1970s, and started jogging in 1972. But I was wearing Keds®! I didn't know anything about running and had no one to talk to about it. After about three weeks my ankles were swollen and I had to stop.

A few years later, on March 6, 1977, I tried again because some of my children were running. I went out with my daughters early in the morning. After two weeks they gave it up, but I was HOOKED! My oldest son, Tom, ran track in high school and then competed in college, but was injured. He continues to run as an adult, although he has had to cope with more injuries. A few years ago he ran a 10-miler in 64 minutes. I was impressed!!! My 22-year-old grandson, Tommy Mac, has run, but currently is focused on baseball. He uses his running speed to steal bases!

Fortunately for me I worked with an excellent runner, Sheldon Karlin, who won the New York Marathon in 1972. He encouraged me and took me to a running store to purchase my first pair of shoes. He also introduced me to several of his Central Park Track Club (CPTC) friends.

I started by running one quarter mile around a track. By the third day I ran a mile. Once I got to two miles I started running on the road. My first race was a 10K in Central Park on June 4, 1977, just three months after I started running!! Sheldon talked me into entering that race. I kept telling him that I didn't run fast enough, but he convinced me that I could do it. When I finished (about an 8:30 pace) and was given a medal I thought, "Oh my goodness, I must be an athlete." My second race was a half marathon in Princeton in September that year. A couple of weeks later I ran a 20K in North Jersey. I don't remember what town, but recall that I was tired. I probably did not rest enough after the half marathon. Then I injured my knees—didn't know that I needed new shoes!!

When I was ready to run my first marathon, Jane Killion, a notable runner and a member of the CPTC, told me about the Avon International Marathon that was being held on March 19, 1978. I had planned to do a March marathon in Monmouth, New Jersey, but was talked into doing the one in Atlanta. My time was 4:01:58. In September I went home to Chicago to run a marathon there. Then New York in October; Jersey Shore in December; Miami in January 1979; the Prevention Marathon in Bethlehem, Pennsylvania, in March; and the Penn Relays in Philadelphia in April. That was six marathons in seven months! In 1991 I ran the Marine Corps Marathon in 3:36, a week later the Atlantic City Marathon in 4:03, and three weeks later the Baltimore Road Runners Marathon in Gunpowder Falls State Park in 3:45. I have run the Boston Marathon 10 times. My fastest marathon was a 3:16:35 at Jersey Shore in 1978. It took a couple more years for me to realize that I was not national-class.

I have a competitive side, possibly from growing up in a large family. In 1990 I ran the Long Beach Island 18-Mile Run in about 2:27 and came in second in my age group. The woman who won my age group ran 2:22. The following year I ran a 2:17 to win the age group and break the age-group record. The next year someone broke my record. That's how it goes.

In addition to my long-distance running, I qualified for the National Senior Olympics in 1992 and competed in Baton Rouge in 1993. I ran three events and won gold in my age group for the 1500.

Sheldon Karlin was my role model. He was 13 years younger than me and very casual in his appearance and personality, but a very competitive runner. In 1972, he was a student at the University of Maryland and had requested scholarship money. His request was denied, so he quit the cross-country team and went to New York City to run the marathon—and won it! When the first Trevira Twosome, a 10-miler, was run, Sheldon asked me to be his partner. I had the age and he had the time. He ran a 51:05 and we won first in our age category.

Another person I admire is Kathrine Switzer. She was the first woman to run the Boston Marathon with a number (1967), and was hassled by Jock Semple, the race director, who tried to remove her when he saw that she was female. However, her hammer-throwing boyfriend took care of him, and she was able to complete the race. Kathrine Switzer organized races for women, and she was in Atlanta for the Avon International Marathon, my first. Before the race she advised us to drink liquid at every water stop, and encouraged us to take the electrolyte replacement with glucose drink that would be offered on the course. And that is what I did and continue to do today, even on training runs. The drink, developed by Bill Gookin, a marathon runner, was called Gookinaid (now Vitalyte®).

I keep yearly running logs; however, regretfully, I disposed of the first 10 years during a move. I have them from 1987 to the present, although they aren't as neat as I would like them to be. I also have a list of all my marathons, but did not keep all the times.

I belong to several running clubs in New Jersey: Pineland Striders, South Jersey AC, Jersey Shore Running Club, and Freehold Area Running Club. I was also a member of the Philadelphia Northeast Road Runners.

My last marathon was my fourth Marine Corps Marathon in 2003. It was my slowest marathon, yet I won first place in my age category. Previously I had received two second place and one third place at Marine Corps. So first place was a nice way to end my marathon career. I stopped running marathons because my body could no longer handle the training for a full marathon. Since 2003, I had been running at least two half marathons a year until very recently.

In 1991, at the age of 54 when I was very well trained, I ran a South Jersey Athletic Club (SJAC) three-loop race at Cooper River (10.95 miles) at a 7:46 pace. This year, I ran one 3.65-mile loop at an 11:35 pace. I talked recently with some of the group I trained with 20 years ago, and reminded them of how fast we were then. The slowing is inevitable. Why do some runners stop racing as they get older? It could be injuries, or it could simply be embarrassment at being very slow.

Training Schedule

During my peak training years I averaged about 40 miles a week. My highest weekly mileage was 67 in the mid-1980s. Altogether, I have run 50 marathons, so each marathon was, in a sense, training for the next. I also did long runs of up to 20 miles, sometimes back-to-back. I was working full-time during this period, so I didn't do much but work and run.

My cross-training, for the most part, is done at the Hamilton YMCA and includes Pilates, yoga, spinning, circuit-training classes, and some upper-body workouts on machines.

Injuries

I've had some injuries. In 1981, after Boston, I developed shin splints. I bought a Schwinn® bicycle to ride while recovering. In 1992, I was probably running too much and had a pelvic stress fracture. A stress fracture means six weeks of no running. Instead, I learned how to swim, something that is really good for a runner. I was taught how to breathe while swimming and got up to a mile. Then I competed in two sprint triathlons, one in 1993 and one in 1994. A friend gave me a racing bike she wasn't using. I thought if I could complete a triathlon, I would really be an athlete. I was last out of the water, last off the bike, but I picked many off on the run.

Due to a back injury last November brought on by doing heavy-duty house-work, I was unable to run a half marathon this last spring. I have a herniated disk and stenosis. I ran a 34:25 5K last week in spite of this; I'd like to get to 34, which would be an age-graded 70 percent. I've had some treatment including physical therapy for the back injury, and feel I'm getting better.

Diet

My diet varies, but usually I have fresh produce every day and a Lean Cuisine® meal. Also I eat a lot of low-fat yogurt, which satisfies my desire for sweets. I put low-fat Cool Whip on the yogurt. And instead of cereal in the morning, I have a banana and some plain soft Jewish rye bread. I take a lot of vitamins and supplements: iron, B12, calcium with vitamin D, cod liver tabs, glucosamine, chondroitin, ginkgo biloba, and cranberry tabs. I spread them out during the day.

Current Goals

I am still hoping to run the Seaside Half Marathon mid-October. But if I'm not able to do it, perhaps I can run a 15K that will be held in Delaware at the beginning of October. And I just found out about the New Jersey Senior Olympics, which will be held next year. I will be 75 (a new age group) in 2012, and will perhaps participate in some track events.

Benefits

I continue to run and race for all the benefits: fitness, good health, stress relief, the feeling of accomplishment, and the opportunities for socializing. I have boxes of trophies that I received for my age-group awards. Now I live near a park, a nice place to run. Very important to me is having the opportunity to just be alone and think things through, whatever they might be.

In the Future

I am planning to continue running for many more years. And I will also continue to participate in the many excellent classes that are offered at my local YMCA.

I already decided that when I get to the point where I can no longer race, I will volunteer for some races just to socialize with the running community. I'm grateful for the years of running I've had and the people I've met. I feel proud of my accomplishments.

MARY HARADA
Newton, Massachusetts

September 2011

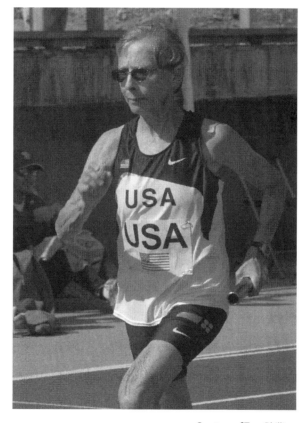

Courtesy of Tom Phillips

Age: 76
Started running: Age 34
Current training per week: 15–20 miles
Long run: 8 miles
Best race: Mile, age-group world record, W70: 7:12:59 at the 2006 USA Masters Indoor Track & Field Championships

I found success in the middle distances and began setting age-group records. My first, a world record in the 70–74 division, was in 2006 in the mile, running 7:12 at the USA Masters Indoor Track & Field Championships in Boston. June and July 2010 were particularly memorable: a 75–79 world and American record for the mile at a race in Concord, Massachusetts, on my 75th birthday, followed by a trip to the Hayward Classic in Eugene, Oregon, where about ten days later I lowered the mark.

Early Years and Family

I was born in Boston and grew up in Newton, Massachusetts. My father was Professor of History at Boston University. Although my mother didn't work after marriage, she earned her M.A. degree in geology from Boston University.

In high school, I played field hockey, basketball, and softball. In college, although there were no sports for women, I played for the Boston Field Hockey Association and joined a fencing club that practiced in my college gym. I also did a lot of biking and hiking in the White Mountains.

I am a retired community-college professor, married with two sons, two daughters-in-law, and one granddaughter.

Getting Started

I began running after graduating with my Ph.D. from Boston University and starting my first full-time college teaching job. A good friend showed me Kenneth Cooper's book, *Aerobics* (Bantam Books, 1969), and the exercise program she was using—I thought it was a good idea to do something, and running did not require finding someone to play tennis or acquiring a lot of equipment. Besides not wanting to gain weight, I wanted to exercise, as I always felt better when I was in decent physical shape—it's good for stress relief.

Although I started running in the fall of 1969, I did not enter a race until sometime in 1977. My first race was a local fun run in the next town, where I ran Saturday mornings with a group of friends. Those Saturday runs ranged in length from two to 10 miles (run on a two-mile loop). We'd start from the house of a friend, Rick Bayko, a longtime Newburyport runner and very good marathoner back in the day. Rick published *Yankee Runner* magazine. This was a mimeograph publication, typed and printed (remember typewriters?) in the days before *Runner's World*. It listed race results. For races, we would get a chintzy prize of a pencil with "Yankee Runner" stamped on it. While Rick stopped the magazine after *Runner's World* started, the Yankee Runner name lives on. It's also the name of a running store he opened in Newburyport 31 years ago.

The first race where I recall my time was over Heartbreak Hill in Newton. I was surprised that I ran a 8:30 per mile pace—and thought, "Hmm, if I trained I could get faster."

Progression

And I did get faster for a few years. In 1979, I ran the Boston Marathon in a time of about 3:30. Unfortunately, I was listed as DNF—the timers did not record my finish. But I had a witness: Fred Brown, longtime president of the North Medford Club (NMC), saw me finish from the NMC hotel-room window overlooking the finish line. The club gave me a big trophy for being the first NMC woman finisher (and only woman in the club to run the race—there were only two women members), and I have a photo of me crossing the railroad bridge, just before Kenmore Square, which is near the finish.

As a child I was greatly impressed with Fanny Blankers-Koen—the Dutch Olympian "housewife" who won four gold medals in the 1948 Olympics. I remember seeing her run in a newsreel and thinking how great she was. After I started going to road races—and there were few women running in the 1970s, and even fewer masters women—I met Sara Mae Berman, who had won Boston three times (1969–71), setting the course record once. With her husband Larry, she founded Cambridge Sports Union, which I joined in the early 1980s. Another woman who impressed me was Miki Gorman, the Japanese American, who won Boston in 1974 and again in 1977 (and who also held the course record of 2:47).

I used to run the 10-mile Yankee Homecoming race in Newburyport (unconnected with Rick Bayko, although he ran it many times) back in the late 1970s and early 1980s. When I started running that race, they gave prizes to the first X number of finishers—who were all male, of course. Eventually they started giving awards to women too.

As I hit my 50s and 60s, I got slower. I ran six marathons before deciding that, if I wanted to get faster, I needed to focus on speed and run shorter distances. In time I took up running track and cross-country, which I much prefer to long road races. I usually train three times a week, rarely four.

I joined the North Medford Club (NMC) around 1977, and then Cambridge Sports Union (CSU), because they had more women members than the two in NMC. CSU had weekly track practices, which I enjoyed. In 1985 I joined Liberty Athletic Club, a women's club, for the number of masters runners. I have been its president for the past 10 years, and I volunteer occasionally—but not as often as I should.

I have run every distance from 200 meters to the marathon. These days I rarely race anything longer than a 6K. Almost all my racing is on the track or cross-country; road racing involves too much pounding for me, but I miss the social aspect of it. I now am what is called a "middle distance" runner. I prefer the 1500, mile, 3K, and 5K distances, but I also race the 400 and the 800 meters occasionally.

I found success in the middle distances and began setting age group records. My first, a world record in the 70–74 division, was in 2006 in the mile, running 7:12 at the USA Masters Indoor Track & Field Championships in Boston. June and July 2010 were particularly memorable: a 75–79 world and American record for the mile at a race in Concord, Massachusetts, on my 75th birthday, followed by a trip to the Hayward Classic in Eugene, Oregon, where about ten days later I lowered the mark. My brother traveled out to Eugene to watch and cheer me on. Then, at the National Masters Outdoor Track meet in Sacramento, July 2010, I set American records for the 5K (26:55) and the 1500 (7:31).

Injuries

Whether caused by the wrong shoes or some other biomechanical problem, anyone who runs on a regular basis has injuries. I am no exception. Most of the time, I have treated myself—and have managed to recover eventually despite the fact that I kept on running. The lesson I learned is that when you start limping while running, but continue running, you will add to the original problem. I have an excellent massage therapist whom I see on a regular basis. And when I need something more, I go to a local acupuncturist who is very good at treating my many aches and pains.

Finding Time

Because I am retired, though, finding time to run is no problem—when I was teaching, I trained during a break between classes, or right after I got home from work and before my kids got off the school bus.

Diet

I don't have a special diet—no fads, no vegan, no vegetarian, etc. My diet is influenced by my Japanese husband. We eat a lot of white rice, which is not exactly a health food, and not a lot of meat. We do not serve dessert with meals, not because of weight control; we just do not have that habit, probably because it is not the custom in Japan. We do have sweets in the house; they are just not a regular part of our daily diet. The only supplements I take are calcium and fish oil (which does wonders for dry skin in the winter). I feel that, because I run, I do not need additional supplements.

Shoes

I buy my shoes at the New Balance® Outlet in Boston and have worn only New Balance® (except for cross country and track shoes) for close to 40 years. For roads, I prefer a lightweight and flexible, but not minimalist, shoe. I wear a spikeless cross-country shoe on the track—until recently, the Nike® Jana. Unfortunately, shoe companies get caught up with fads—either overengineering their shoes trying to cure whatever foot weirdness they think you have, or trying to make you run barefoot. The fashion now is "minimalist"—well, fine if you have really good feet that do not need any support. But for the vast majority of runners, wearing these shoes is a great way to damage your feet.

Current Goals

My current goals are to slow down as little as possible and to stay as injury free as possible, although age makes this a challenge.

Benefits

I am not sure what expected benefits I thought I would get from running. It has become a habit; it is what I do. Running keeps my weight in check, it helps me stay healthy, and it has been a great stress reliever. Some unexpected benefits include the great people I have met at races and track meets around the world—the opportunities to travel for a sport I enjoy, and meet others who enjoy it as well. What I most like about running is that little equipment is needed. I can do it just about anywhere.

In the Future

Besides running, I enjoy travel, reading, using all my electronic gadgets, and participating in local politics—strictly town stuff: School Committee, Board of Health, Finance Committee, and now the local Housing Authority. All of those except Finance Committee were elected positions.

I am still running at 76 and hope to be able to continue for many years. I like to joke that I will be running to my funeral.

CAROL MONTGOMERY
Treasure Island, Florida

December 2011

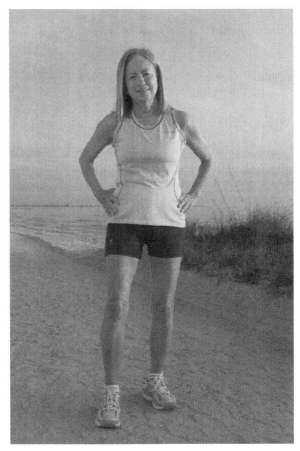

Courtesy of Mike MacKay

Age: 76

Started running: Age 43

Current training per week: 20 miles running and slogging

Long run: 7 miles now; 8.4 miles for 30 years

Best race: Boston Marathon at age 70, 5:05:35, second in age group

One of my most memorable moments of the NYC marathon was at the starting line—way back in the pack. It was unusual for 50-year-old women to run marathons at the time (1985) and I was, you could say, "full of it." There was a woman standing next to me who said that she was 70. I thought she was crazy. Twenty years later I found myself on the starting line of the Boston Marathon.

Early Years and Family

I was born and grew up in Davenport, Iowa, with three younger siblings: one sister and two brothers. My parents played golf. My father had polio as a child; the lingering effects limited his ability to play many sports. As a grade-schooler I learned to swim, and remember doing the high jump and triple jump in middle school. I was very interested in gymnastics, and attended classes at a local organization. But the training was limited and there were no competitions. I had the ideal body type for gymnastics—short, small-boned and thin—and would have loved the opportunity to excel at it.

I went to a Catholic girls' high school that had no athletic programs. I played golf at the local country club, then went to Bryn Mawr, a women's college in suburban Philadelphia that required regular gym classes and passing a swimming test (not a problem). I remember taking fencing. There was an active field hockey program that did not interest me at all.

Everyone smoked at the time. My parents smoked; I smoked. I married a man right after college who smoked a lot—I never got above half a pack a day. I stopped smoking (several times) in my mid-30s but still sometimes had the urge when I was under a lot of stress. Running cured that.

I had one child, a son. Divorced when I was in my mid-30s, I obtained a master's degree, then went to work as an information scientist for an innovative Philadelphia company. During one summer in Iowa my father taught my son, David, to play golf and he became an excellent golfer. He was captain of his high-school golf team and even played in the U.S. Amateur one year.

Getting Started

I enrolled in a doctoral program when David went to college in 1976, and started working part-time so I could complete my dissertation. This was an extremely stressful time—I would wake up early in the morning and not be able to get back to sleep, and even worse, was beginning to gain weight. I had become aware of running as an adult sport from two coworkers who were running together in the morning before work. So I decided to go outside and give it a try. I bought a book about running which—REALLY!—cautioned that too much might be bad for a woman's reproductive system. I ran a little, walked a little, until one day a younger woman from the apartment complex joined me. We ran together (about half a mile, I think) to the track of a local boys' prep school, around the track and back.

I obtained my doctoral degree in 1979 and moved to Lexington, Kentucky, to teach at the University of Kentucky. I continued running around my neighborhood in the early morning. There was another faculty member who ran, and he invited me to go with him and his wife to a running club that met on Saturday mornings. It was a lovely place; the clubhouse was in a building that was part of a horse farm. We all ran various distances on the roads around the gorgeous bluegrass countryside, and then came back to the clubhouse for coffee and food. I ran two miles; then, one day I missed a turn and ended up running six miles. That was a life-changing moment. I continued doing the six-mile distance and ran my first race, a 10K, in the spring. I was basically clueless about what to expect, and have no idea what my time was. But I won my age group and came home with a huge, ugly trophy. The name of the race was Run Kentucky Run and I still have the trophy. That was another life-changing moment.

Progress

When I moved back to Philadelphia the following summer for a job as a medical library director, I discovered that there were many races in the area on weekends and started going to them. I began to make friends in the running community. One told me that "you can always run three times your daily distance," so I picked it up to four miles a day and started running "the loop" on weekends. The loop is an 8.4-mile trek from the Philadelphia Art Museum along the east side of the Schuylkill River to the bridge in East Falls, and back on the west side.

That year I ran many 5Ks and 10Ks and my first half marathon, the Philadelphia Distance Run. The next spring I did the Broad Street 10 Mile Run, the largest race in Philadelphia at that time. I usually placed in my age group in the smaller races and Broad Street, but not the Distance Run until I turned 70. In 1983, one of my brothers was running the New York City Marathon and wanted me to run him in. I did. It was spectacular, an incredible crowd. I was 48 then, and decided to run the New York City Marathon the year I turned 50.

I also changed jobs that year and bought a condominium right across the street from the Philadelphia Art Museum. It seemed like a perfect place for a runner—the sidewalk along the river for training, and most of the races in

Philadelphia started near the museum. For training, I followed religiously a six-month day-by-day schedule that I had found in a magazine. Since the NYC Marathon was at the end of October, this meant a lot of mornings and nights running in the dark. I remember one morning when I got up at 4 a.m. in order to finish a long run in time to go to work. Unfortunately, the city was not the safest place for a woman to be alone in the dark. I survived, but one female runner in that area did not several years later. I ran New York in 4:23, 20 seconds faster than my younger brother two years earlier! The last 10 miles of the marathon were agonizing. I decided I had marathon bragging rights and would never do another one.

One of my most memorable moments of the NYC marathon was at the starting line—way back in the pack. It was unusual for 50-year-old women to run marathons at the time and I was, you could say, "full of it." There was a woman standing next to me who said that she was 70. I thought she was crazy.

Twenty years later, I found myself on the starting line of the Boston Marathon. During the years in between I almost always ran Broad Street and the Distance Run. The Distance Run was my life check—if I finished, I was okay. Fortunately, I joined a running group coached by a former elite runner, Mike Patterson. The group met every Tuesday night at 6:30 p.m. at a boathouse just west of the art museum. The members were young, old, fast, slow, and from all walks of life. Everyone was friendly and supportive. I was one of the oldest and slowest, but it didn't matter. We did speed work—I didn't understand how important that was for me until I stopped doing it 15 years later when I moved from Philadelphia. I learned so much from Mike and the group.

In the spring, all the group's runners' thoughts turned to Boston. Who had qualified? Where? Who was going? When they returned, how did they do? When I turned 60 I checked my qualifying time and quickly decided I had no chance. The qualifying time was faster than I had run the New York City Marathon at 50. Then, about five years later, due mainly to the efforts of Dr. Walter Bortz, founder of the Fifty-Plus Fitness Association, qualifying times for older runners were raised substantially. As a 70-year-old woman I would only need to run a qualifying marathon under five hours. This seemed doable, since at 68 I was still running the half marathon in about 2:15 without any special training.

So I decided to give it a shot. I planned to qualify at the Philadelphia Marathon, which had the dual advantage of being one of the fastest qualifiers, and starting in front of the art museum, almost at my front door. This time I had a coach, Mike Patterson. He gave me a month-by-month plan that included double long workouts on weekends. I was still working full-time at a demanding job, so my life became: eat, train, work, sleep. All was going well until I got an iliotibial band (ITB) injury three weeks before the marathon. After putting so much time and effort into the training, I felt depressed. I couldn't run, so I swam and water-jogged, and used the elliptical for several hours on weekends.

But I had registered, it was a beautiful morning, the marathon start was right out the door, and I knew the course well, so I knew I could get home easily when I had to quit. I was amazed that I could run without pain. I was under two and a half hours at the 14-mile point, which comes back by the start. I knew I was under my qualifying time, with a cushion, and I was so happy I felt no pain. This was the first and last time I've had a runner's high. The pain came back at mile 24, so I walked until I saw the clock, and then ran, again feeling nothing. My time was 4:52:44. I had qualified for Boston!

Next, the problem became staying in shape for Boston. I followed the same rigorous training plan, worked one day a week with a Pilates instructor, and added swimming once or twice a week. My son, who was 46, qualified so he could run with me. He and my daughter-in-law and two grandsons all made the trip. This was 2005, after the chip was used, but when everyone still started at noon. The weather was great, helpful during the four-plus-hour wait in Hopkinton before the start. It took us almost 18 minutes after the gun went off to get to the starting line. My goal had been a Boston Marathon finisher's medal, which you receive only if you finish under six hours. My finishing time was 5:05:21. I was the second of four women over 70 to finish. I came home with much more than a medal.

After 70, my speed declined rapidly. So did my motivation to train for long races. It took me almost an hour longer to run the Marine Corps Marathon a year and a half after Boston (5:54). My last marathon, Medoc (in some of France's most famous vineyards), took over six hours; it was great fun, though, for the scenery, the wine, the food, and the slow, party atmosphere. I have run a few half marathons since, but as my half times went over three hours, I decided to limit my races to shorter distances.

After I retired, I volunteered to be a trainer for the Team in Training and the Philadelphia-area Galloway training group. Both organizations aim to turn nonrunners into runners, usually working toward a marathon as a goal. They hold increasingly long group runs on Saturdays, offer guidance on what to run on weekdays, and provide needed general advice. My reasoning was that I could help with pacing—most new runners try to go too fast, then cannot continue. I had the endurance to stay with the young, new runners on the long runs. I did this until I moved out of the Philadelphia area. Now, I sometimes volunteer at local races when I'm not running.

Training Schedule

I keep logs of my training and my races in spreadsheets. I track training miles, and for races, distance, time, minutes per mile, and place in my age group. I also note cross-training activities such as spinning, time on an elliptical machine, stretching, core strength training, and use of free weights. I stretch, do strength training almost daily, and lift free weights three times a week. I've decreased my running miles and increased the cross-training as I've gotten older. I can maintain my weight with this routine.

Injuries

I did not have any running injuries until I was 60. Then, due probably to using old running shoes, I developed plantar fasciitis. That cleared up in a few weeks with rest. So did the ITB band pull and a partial hamstring tear caused by too much hard downhill running. Now I wear well-cushioned neutral shoes that I rotate regularly and fit with Power Bounce™ inserts.

Diet

My diet is generally healthy with an emphasis on fish, chicken, and yogurt for protein; whole grains, fruits, and vegetables. I usually eat spaghetti before races, although it is not necessary for 5Ks. My "cheating" consists of a glass of wine with dinner and a small dessert after. I take a multivitamin, calcium, and fish oil. When I was running long distances I used an energy drink and power bars.

Benefits

When I started running, my goals were weight maintenance and stress reduction. I've achieved those goals and benefited in so many other ways. Until this past year I had the same energy level as in my 20s. I look much younger than my age and have good overall health. Unexpectedly, I have made many good friends in the running community, including my partner, an outstanding runner in his 70s.

I like to combine racing with travel. We have gone on several organized running cruises to the Caribbean and Alaska with Cruise to Run, managed by a Canadian company. Other trips include the Medoc Marathon with Marathon Tours, the Amsterdam Marathon on our own, and in November 2011 the Havana

Marabana—notable for having over a thousand runners in five distances (5K, 10K, 15K, half marathon, marathon) all starting at once AND having NO porta potties or other bathroom facilities at the start. Still a neat race and fun.

Current Goals

I had expected that my Boston Marathon at 70 would be a "last hurrah," and that I would slow down, eventually walk and run, and then just walk. I just didn't see women in their 70s running, and I was okay with that at the time. However, after Boston, I continued running and racing, albeit more slowly, until I was 75.

Then, I developed severe sciatica caused by a bulging, herniated disc in my back. I could not exercise at all during the acute phase—about two months. When I tried to get back to running I could only run short spurts, then slog—my feet did not get off the ground. I had back surgery to fix the disc, and tried to run again after a month. It was harder than when I first started running. One minute run, one minute walk, two minutes run, one minute walk, working up to the point where I was jogging half miles alternating with walking 100 meters. I now "run" 5Ks in about 40 minutes. At this level I can participate in races with my partner when he runs 5Ks or longer races. That is my current goal. I'm not optimistic that my times will improve further. If I can't participate in races, I'll volunteer.

ZANDRA MOBERG PRICE
July 21, 2011

Philadelphia, Pennsylvania

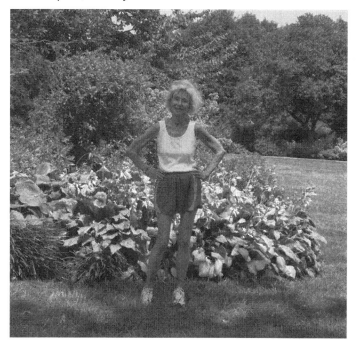

Age: 76
Started running: Age 35
Current training per week: 20 miles
Long run: 10–11 miles
Best race: The Philadelphia Distance Run at age 66, my
first half marathon

Sometimes I run when I visit my mother in the Poconos and then I enjoy the sights in my hometown, now so changed, or in the lovely woods along a creek. I have run in London, Prague, Atlanta, Washington, Albuquerque, Anchorage, Colorado, Utah, North and South Carolina, the Jersey shore. I always take running gear when I travel, just in case

Early Years and Family

I was born in Stroudsburg, Pennsylvania, in the Pocono Mountains and grew up there. I'm half Czech and half English/Scotch-Irish, a mutt like most Americans. In 2001, right after 9/11, I visited Prague, ran there a few times, and learned to speak a little Czech. As a child and teenager I was terrible at sports. I did enjoy running, but track for girls did not exist at my school. I did a lot of hiking in the Poconos, and still do when I can.

I attended Swarthmore College for two years, finishing a bachelor's degree in history at the University of Pennsylvania years later after my children were born. I had moved to Powelton Village in Philadelphia, where I met and married my husband. We started our family there, a daughter and a son. Powelton Village was a memorably happening place to be in the 1960s.

I have three grandchildren. The oldest is a sophomore at the University of South Carolina. She runs as part of her fitness program there. My son ran in school and may get back to it, but right now he is too busy heading a laboratory doing cancer research at Emory University and being an involved father. My daughter works hard on environmental issues and does more walking than running. My husband, Al, doesn't run anymore but I have noticed that when we have to make a dash for the bus, he is way faster than me.

Getting Started

I began running during a very stressful period in my life. I had left my first husband and moved back home to Stroudsburg. I found that running in place in front of the TV helped my shattered nerves. That led to jogging for a mile on a two-lane road near my house. People on their front porches used to yell to ask who was chasing me. That was 1970, before the first running boom. I was not aware of serious running. Then I heard about a jogging group at East Stroudsburg University and went to see the coach, Herb Weber, who encouraged me to join. I only went to the group a few times because the workouts were on a track and I didn't like using one—not nearly as interesting as the road—but I was eternally grateful for the support. An important thing I learned from Herb was that it was not crazy to run, quite the contrary.

I remember being impressed by a movie that Herb showed us about a depressed man in New York who decided to run to commit suicide—his plan was to just run and run until he collapsed. He ran and ran and you can guess what happened—his depression was cured and he became a runner.

After a year the children and I moved back to Philadelphia. I happened to meet a young couple who were joggers. The guy told me, "Don't just run a mile, try four miles." I was a little skeptical but it worked. I was then a single parent, trying to do the best possible job raising two young children, working, and plodding away part-time at graduate school in library science at Drexel University. That didn't leave much time for running; I just went when I could to the track at my children's school.

My divorce was difficult and protracted. I moved to Florida for nine months, where my mother was living, to get away from it all. I worked in the Li'l General convenience store, went swimming in the Gulf, and ran. One of the customers told me about a 10K race there and I signed up—my first race. I kept looking anxiously behind me to see if I was the last one. I wasn't, but there were lots of people ahead of me. I still look behind me in races.

Running for me is a solitary activity. I don't run with a partner, but I recognize other runners, and I will often wave or speak to them. Sometimes young women, or even men, tell me that I'm an inspiration or that they want to be like me when they get old. That inspires me too. I would advise anyone who wants to try running to just do it and keep going. If you are tired after one mile, you will not be more tired after four, really. Keep going—that is, if you enjoy it. People have to like the exercise they are doing or they won't do it. And here is important advice that Herb Weber passed on to us in the group so long ago: "Listen to your body."

Progression

I finished my master's degree at last; the children went off to college and all I was doing was working, so I was able to start running regularly. I had a boyfriend who was really dedicated. We ran in 10Ks together and once had our picture taken with Grete Waitz. Last I heard, he wasn't running anymore because of knee problems. He was one of many people I used to run with who always told me to run faster, that I wasn't pushing hard enough, that I could do better. I ignored them and just kept going at my own lackadaisical speed while they forged ahead. I think it's significant that all of them have stopped running, due mostly to their knees giving out.

When I got to my 50s there were very few women my age running 10Ks. Incredibly, many times I'd just have to show up to win my age group. It was definitely a lift for previously noncompetitive me to win prizes. Things have changed since then. Now there are far fewer 10Ks and many more women in their 50s running. Age-group awards used to be huge statues of runners. I have a box of those. Now many of the awards are medals or nice glass sculptures.

I usually run two or three races a year. I ran my first 10-mile race, Broad Street, in the 1980s. My boyfriend had done it one year and I thought, "I can do that." I have done Broad Street fairly regularly over the years and usually win something in my age group. Once, at the awards ceremony, as I was picking up my statue, the woman who was giving them out commented icily that my time was slow. It was, but this was an age-group award, after all.

By 1990 I was working at the Free Library of Philadelphia and living in an apartment in the Art Museum area that was near both my job and the Schuylkill River. There is a wonderful path along the river, paralleling Kelly Drive on one side and Martin Luther King Jr. Drive on the other. The entire loop—from the museum, over a bridge, and back to the museum—is 8.4 miles. It's a beautiful and very popular place to run, walk, or bike—even in the winter, when the city keeps it well-plowed. Over these 20 years It has been great to watch the advance in racial diversity on Kelly Drive. In 1990 I saw very few African Americans running there, and just about no African-American women. Now in 2011, when I go out in the morning, there are sometimes more people of color—including lots of women—than white people.

In 2001 I went to hear Amby Burfoot speak at Whole Foods in Philadelphia. I told him (timidly) that I had done 10-mile races and I asked him if he thought I could do a half marathon. He immediately said, "Sure." I used to admire the people in the Philadelphia Distance Run, a half marathon that includes the "loop," and now I was actually going to be one of them! I have run the Distance Run nearly every year since and, as I recall, placed in my age group in all but one.

I rarely run 5Ks, but a couple of years ago I did one to benefit the local NPR radio station. I was 74 and the age groups ended at 60-plus, so I didn't win anything—got beat by a woman in her early 60s, I think. It didn't seem quite fair. Made me admit then that I am more competitive than I thought. I have kept a somewhat haphazard file of most of my race results and race numbers.

I have had little adventures while running. About seven years ago, near the Strawberry Mansion Bridge on Kelly Drive, I saw a man sprawled out on the hill in the trees across the busy street. A blue knit hat covered most of his face and head. It was troubling. Later I stopped at the police station and almost apologetically told them about the man, saying it was probably nothing. The next day I was surprised to spot an article in the paper about the police finding a body on the Drive that had been reported by a jogger. I called it my moment of anonymous fame. He had been shot in the head, hence the blue hat.

Training

I walk a lot and go to the gym once or twice a week. There I do upper-body work, because running works the lower body and I'd like to have better-toned shoulders. I read a long time ago that you shouldn't run every day. I try to get out every other day. When I am training for a half marathon, my weekly distance goes up to 24 miles a week, and the long run to 13 miles.

Injuries

I had a maddening injury two years ago that kept me from running for almost three months. It was severe pain behind the knee if I tried to run. I saw several doctors. None of them diagnosed anything and it finally went away. One MRI technician said that I had a baker's cyst, and that could explain the pain. Otherwise, I have not been troubled much by injuries, although twice I injured my hamstring trying to go up steep hills as fast as I could. I feel lucky that when I trip and fall on my knees, they don't break. I've never had knee pain, although I've fallen many times and have nasty scars all over my knees. I've had unsightly varicose veins for decades, but so far they don't bother me physically.

Finding Time

As a retiree I'm heavily involved in volunteer activities. When other activities conflict with running, I usually give priority to these other things. I don't usually go for a long run on Sundays because I might get back too late for Quaker meeting. I volunteer as a guide at a Quaker meetinghouse once a week, and right now work with anti-fracking and anti-war groups. One is the Granny Peace Brigade Philadelphia. To protest the Iraq war in 2006, 11 of us staged a sit-in at an army recruiting center and were arrested.

Diet

I make an effort to know a lot about nutrition. I subscribe to the *Nutrition Action Health Letter* from the Center for Science and the Public Interest to keep up-to-date on new discoveries. I try to drink lots of milk because osteoporosis runs in my family. I am mostly vegetarian and eat very few sweets. I take calcium religiously and plenty of antioxidants (not knowing if they do any good, but I don't want to take any chances). Research data indicate that resveratrol, an ingredient in red wine, may prolong life and delay age-related illnesses. Who knows? Anyhow, my husband and I drink red wine.

I drink only water during long runs or races because the sports drinks make me nauseous. The last time I did the Distance Run I felt dizzy at the end, and it dawned on me that it might be caused by low blood sugar. I eat very little before a race. I'm going to start taking power bars when I'm doing long-distance.

Current Goals

My current goal is to run the Philadelphia Distance Run this September, and after that to work out more at the gym.

Benefits

I don't focus on time or competing against myself. I am kind of a running dilettante. I do it for fun, for fitness, to get centered. Most important, I pray, meditate, think, figure things out, soul-search. If I don't run for a long time I feel uneasy. The experience along the river is visually wonderful—the trees, the water, the people, even the geese.

There is strong evidence that running protects one from Alzheimer's. That is significant for me because my poor mother has Alzheimer's and it's not pretty. Sometimes I run when I visit her in a nursing home in the Poconos and then I enjoy the sights in my hometown, now so changed, or in the lovely woods along a creek. I have run in London, Prague, Atlanta, Washington, Albuquerque, Anchorage, Colorado, Utah, North and South Carolina, the Jersey shore. I always take running gear when I travel, just in case.

In the Future

I hope I will still be running in five years, even longer. But if not, that's okay too—it's been a great run.

July 11, 2011

KATHERINE BEIERS
Santa Cruz, California

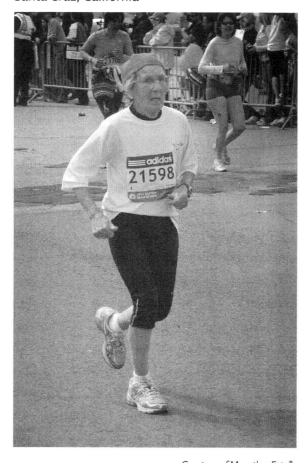

Courtesy of MarathonFoto®

Age: 79
Started running: Age 49
Current training per week: 25–30 miles
Long run: 9–17 miles
Best race: Boston Marathon at age 78, age-group winner and 10 minutes faster than previous year

A memorable race was the Mayo Midnight Marathon in Keno City, Yukon, when I was 68. The race started at midnight in June. Since we were close to the Arctic Circle, it was light all night. Because of the prevalence of black bears in the area, we had car escorts so if a bear appeared we could hop in. At about mile 22 I saw some animals that were too small for bears. Just then a car came up beside me. They identified the animals as a pack of wolves. I would not get in the car; I was so close to the end that I wanted to finish. So, the car escorted me in to a 4:45 finish.

Early Years and Family

I was born into an Irish/German family in Langdon, North Dakota, and grew up there. I went to St. Catherine's University in St. Paul, Minnesota—a Catholic girls' college—and later earned my master's degree in library science at the University of Southern California. I did not participate in sports in high school, college, or afterwards until I started running. Langdon was a very small town with no swimming pool and no tennis courts, but it did have a nine-hole golf course with sand greens. My father played golf, and I played a little while I was in high school.

I was married to a doctor who got his medical degree at the University of Pennsylvania. While we were there, I worked in the Wharton Business School library as a reference librarian and loved it. My husband died in a plane crash when I was 29.

I have two daughters who live with their husbands and children in Portland, Oregon, and a son who lives in San Carlos, California, near San Francisco. They have given me ten grandchildren. Ten of my family members just ran a 5K/10K event, and four of us were on the podium receiving awards! One grandson won the 18-to-21 age division; a granddaughter placed in the 5K, and my son—who is now 51—and I won our age groups. My son is an excellent runner. We usually do marathons together—he always runs Boston when I do. He finishes an hour and a half ahead of me, and then he is at the end cheering me in. That my family members are runners makes me very proud—it is really wonderful. My granddaughter, my daughter, and I have run several half marathons together—it's fun to think of us as three generations running.

I was a librarian for 25 years in the University of Santa Cruz science library, where I had a successful career. I became involved in city issues, served on several City of Santa Cruz commissions, and was elected to City Council from 1989 to 2000 and again in 2008 for a term I am currently serving. I was mayor of Santa Cruz in 1994 and again in 1999–2000. The work as councilmember is fulfilling, although sometimes difficult. It was more fun when we had money to do a lot of important and popular things. Now our energies are focused on what to cut.

Getting Started

When I got close to 50 and was starting to gain weight, I had a yearning to try a sport. About then, time management was receiving a lot of attention among administrators. The university invited a time-management guru to give a talk to faculty and other university personnel. He started by talking about stopping martini lunches, and then went on to say that we needed to "pump our hearts" 12 minutes a day. I thought I could do that. He said that all that was necessary was a 12-minute-per-day cardio workout. That talk was the push I needed. I had wanted to get outdoors, exercise, and enjoy our beautiful park-like campus anyway.

So I went to the campus track and started running. It took me several months to do one mile without stopping. I was so excited I called my three kids, who were in college, and told them that I had run a mile. I never thought I would do two miles! A couple of friends who were good runners told me to get off the track and onto the roads. They wanted me to start with them. At first I could only do half a block with them, but I got better and better. They also told me to get new shoes. About a year later I realized I was doing well and liked the physical rewards of running. I would go back to my desk after my running lunch break and have lots of energy. I was really proud of myself. I told my friends that I no longer went to lunch; I went to the track, ran my lunch hour, and then ate something at my desk when I got back. That got me started.

Progression

I started doing 5Ks very soon after I started running, then 10Ks, then half marathons. Two years after I started, I ran my first marathon, Napa Valley in California, and then the first two years of Big Sur, a beautiful marathon. I run about two marathons a year, and I believe I've done close to 30 now. I've run New York five times. I'm doing more trail running and ultra-marathoning now. I've run 15 to 20 50Ks, and three American River 50-milers. The last one was in 2007. I've never tried triathlons—I can't swim.

Another memorable race was the Mayo Midnight Marathon in Keno City, Yukon, when I was 68. I made the 3,000-mile drive with some friends from California. The race started at midnight in June. Since we were close to the Arctic Circle, it was light all night. Because of the prevalence of black bears in the area, we had car escorts so if a bear appeared we could hop in. Before we were allowed to start we had to listen to a half-hour lecture on what to do if you encountered a bear. (Should a reader need to know, you stop, keep your eye on the bear, and back up slowly.) At about mile 22 I saw some animals that were too small for bears. I did what I was told, though, and just then a car came up beside me. They identified the animals as a pack of wolves who intended to cross the road. I would not get in the car; I was so close to the end that I wanted to finish. So, the car escorted me in to a 4:45 finish.

My running friends are all ages, male and female. I have been a member of a local track club ever since its founding. Unfortunately, it is about a 40-minute drive to go to their workouts, so I don't make it often. We have a big (about 15,000) local race the last Sunday in July called the Wharf to Wharf, and the organizers always give me my age as my number. I only know of one other good local female runner about my age—she is just turning 70. There are a few excellent women runners in the Carmel/Monterey area who are in their 70s.

Because I'm well-known in the community, I give talks where I encourage others, especially seniors, to start running. I tell them they can start in their 60s, and many do. I find beginners have a tendency to overdress and then they overheat and become miserable, so I tell them to get dressed, and then take off a layer. Other advice I give to beginners is: Before you start running, decide how far you are going to go. And, don't go farther and don't go less. Sometimes you'll be struggling, but just do it. Sometimes you'll want to go farther, but don't. Take two days a week off.

Training Schedule

Now I'm part of a huge running community. For about 15 years, I ran with two friends at 6 a.m. I have lots of running friends, and so can always find someone to do the distance I want to do. Yesterday I ran 12 miles with 12 women in a state park. The company helps keep me going. No excuses. Now that I'm retired, I don't have to get up at 6 a.m., while all my running friends are much younger and still working. So most of the time I run alone during the week—get my miles in—and run with others on weekends.

When I'm training for a marathon or 50K race, my weekly mileage goes up to 40 or 50 miles, and my long run is 22 miles. My training pace is about 12 minutes per mile. In races, I walk up all the hills and through the aid stations. It works. I ran Boston last April ten minutes faster (11:42 pace) than the previous year, and have not figured out how that happened. When you get older you are supposed to get slower.

Editor's Note: In the last nine years Katherine has run seven Boston Marathons, placing first in her age group four times. She ran 2011 in 4:59:07 and 2010 in 5:09:56, and an amazing 4:43:53 in 2008 at the age of 75. Of the 69 races listed for Katherine on ATHLINKS, she placed first in her age group in 56 and second in 12. Some recent results: Santa Cruz Firecracker 10K at age 78, 1:14:13; Big Sur Half Marathon at age 78, 2:23:51; and American River 50-Miler at age 75, 12:09:13.

I keep a log of my training runs and races. I always write down where I went and how long. I belong to a gym; my coach wanted me to do upper-body work—I just don't like it. I did it for about two weeks and stopped.

Injuries

I've had torn menisuses on both knees, which were operated on, then took off four months per my doctor's orders. During that time, I did water jogging to keep my cardio fitness, making it possible for me to go right back to running once my knees had healed. Now my knees never bother me, and even take me through the 50-mile ultras without a problem.

I remember telling my orthopedic surgeon how lucky I felt that I could continue doing all this running and hiking. He said, "It's not luck, it's your genes." Aren't good genes luck? Bottom line is I don't know how I can keep going when most women can't. I enjoy the running and I'm doing fine. Last week, at 79, I ran a very difficult trail half marathon; we crossed four streams and covered steep descents, which are harder for me now since I know my balance is compromised and I don't want to fall. But I finished with a good time: 3:29.

Diet

I can eat everything. I drink wine with dinner, eat red meat and desserts. I keep my weight at 100 to 102, which is fine for my four-foot, eleven-and-a-half-inch frame. I describe myself as a big eater. My favorite drink after a race is beer. A great recovery drink—revives me instantly. I take no vitamins or supplements and don't use energy drinks. On a long run I drink water and use GU—during a marathon I'll take a GU every hour. On the 50Ks and 50-Milers I take salt tablets too. The aid stations for ultras all have wonderful food that I stop and eat. I developed high blood pressure at about 72, and now take medication for it. My doctor said that if I hadn't been running, it would probably have developed a lot earlier.

Current Goals

I want to run Marine Corps in Washington, D.C., this year and I plan to go back to Boston next year. As an age-group winner, I'm always given a free entry. And my son has qualified too. I'm hoping to do some more ultras, especially 50Ks. I enjoy them. Since they take eight or more hours, it is like being in a park all day. My ultra buddy has moved from the area, and we are trying to find one that would be easy for both of us to travel to. Now that I'm back on City Council, it is harder for me to travel as frequently or for as long periods of time as I did previously.

My other interests besides City Council are travel and visiting my grandchildren, five of whom are in college. I also do multiday hikes. I've just finished a 100-mile, 10-day tour around Mount Blanc in France, Italy, and Switzerland, and with three friends I will be hiking the 250K Cathar Way in southwestern France in September.

In the Future

Right now I have no reason not to keep on running. I like the discipline of the training. The day of the race isn't that big a deal—I've just had a wonderful three months preparing.

LOIS ANN GILMORE
Janesville, Wisconsin

September, 2011

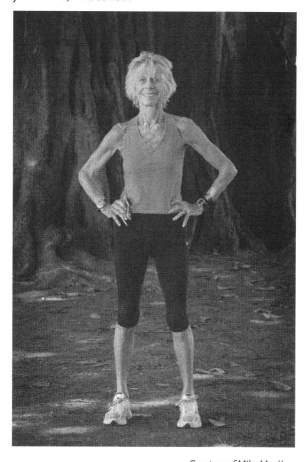

Courtesy of Mike MacKay

Age: 80

Started running: Age 60

Current training per week: Up to 20 miles

Long run: 5 miles, occasionally longer

Best race: Bellin 10K (Green Bay, WI), 55:01. A new age-group world record at 77.

In June of 2011 I was selected to carry the Wisconsin flag in the open-
ing ceremonies of the National Senior Games, also known as the Senior
Olympics, in Houston, Texas. I was the gold medalist in the 80–84 age
group in the 5K and in the 1500 meters, setting Senior Games records. This
was the first time I had competed in these games. Then, on September 1 at
the Huntsman World Senior Games in St. George, Utah, I set four 80–84
age-group records: 4:33 in the 800 meters, 19:12 in the 3000 meters, 9:02
in the 1500 meters, and 30:21 in the 5K.

Early Years and Family

I was born in La Crosse, Wisconsin, in 1930 and grew up on a farm in Onalaska, Wisconsin, near La Crosse. My ancestry is Norwegian/German. The oldest of three sisters, I attended the University of Wisconsin-La Crosse, receiving my B.A. in elementary education in 1951. I taught elementary school in Wisconsin and Illinois. Competitive sports for women were not available in my high school or college, but I was a cheerleader in high school

Wayne Gilmore and I were married in 1955. We have three children, all professionals, and six grandchildren. A retired dentist, Wayne took up running and racing after I did to lose weight and maintain muscle tone. He runs most of the races with me, finishing behind me. That's fine with him. All our children are skiers and runners. My daughters also play tennis, and my son is an Ironman triathlete aiming to complete all nine U.S. Ironman races. All our grandchildren are runners and have been on cross-country and track teams!

I've always been very active as an adult. I've been a downhill and cross-country skier, played tennis and golf, biked recreationally, done strength training with free weights, stretched, and participated in Jazzercise® and other exercise classes. I won many awards in senior tennis tournaments, and coached women's tennis at Beloit College from 1978 to 1980.

Getting Started

While a stay-at-home mom, I found that getting out of the house to jog or walk always improved my mood. I was what you would call a recreational runner. Then, in my late 50s, I had breast cancer and became depressed afterwards. I couldn't play tennis anymore. Running was an important way to cope with the depression. So a few months after my recovery, having walked and jogged on and off for years, I set a goal of running a 5K race. Six months after surgery, I entered a fall road race in Milwaukee and won my age group! This happened in spite of my wearing too many layers of clothing and becoming overheated during the race.

Progression

I decided to run more races, and continued to win my age group. I was motivated to compete more and more and at longer distances. Within a year, I was racing once or twice on most weekends. I race distances from one mile to ten miles, although my most frequent and favorite distance is 5K.

I believe I became a competitive runner so quickly because I was already in shape. I needed to fine-tune my racing with trial and error—e.g., figuring out what clothes to wear, the best shoes for me, and how to pace myself. At first my times improved steadily with each race.

In June of 2011 I was selected to carry the Wisconsin flag in the opening ceremonies of the National Senior Games, also known as the Senior Olympics, in Houston, Texas. I was the gold medalist in the 80–84 age group in the 5K and in the 1500 meters, setting Senior Games records. This was the first time I had competed in these games. Next, on a hot day in late July, I ran the Quad City Times Bix 7—seven hilly miles in Davenport, Iowa—in 73 minutes, a time faster than any other woman over 70. Then on September 1 at the Huntsman World Senior Games in St. George, Utah, I ran eight events, won five, and set four 80–84 age-group records: 4:33 in the 800 meters, 19:12 in the 3000 meters, 9:02 in the 1500 meters, and 30:21 in the 5K.

I keep a meticulous log of my runs and races so I know I have run over 1,200 races, nearly always winning my age group and winning 95 percent of the races if the runners were ranked on the basis of age-graded scores. Mine are consistently over 90 percent.

Editor's Note: Lois Ann's accomplishments after the age of 70 are truly amazing. A short list:

2003: Inducted into the Janesville, Wisconsin Hall of Fame

Age-group records at the Bix 7 (Davenport, Iowa): 70–74, 75–79, 80 plus

2006 and 2007: No. 1 USA Track & Field female runner 75 and over

2007: USA Track & Field Masters Runner of the Year

2008: USA Track & Field Outstanding Athlete of the Year for age division F75

2008 Philadelphia Sports Writers Association gave Lois the Most Courageous Athlete of the Year

2009: Named by Running Times magazine as the top female runner 75–79

2011: Age-group records (80-84) for the 1500 meters and 5K at the National Senior Games (Houston, Texas)

2011: Four age-group records at the Huntsman World Senior Games (St. George, Utah)

I enjoyed the social aspects of skiing, tennis, golf, and biking, so it was natural that I joined running clubs. I belong to the Chicago Area Runners Association (CARA), where I was the first a Hall of Fame inductee; Badgerland Striders; Fox Lake Runners; and the Lisle, Illinois, Runners Club. I read four national running magazines: *Runner's World, Running Times, National Masters News,* and *Women's Running,* plus several regional publications like *Florida Race Place.* We spend part of the winter in Florida.

My role models are Grete Waitz and Joan Benoit Samuelson because of their determination to be the best.

Training Schedule

Currently I train two to three days a week, with runs of three to five miles if I have races on weekends. I usually train during the day, outside around my neighborhood in good weather, often on the Ice Age Trail next to where I live or at the high school track. If the weather is bad I run on the track at the local athletic club. I stretch every other day. I lifted free weights for many years but recently was advised to stop because of sore muscles. One thing I would change about my earlier training is knowing when to take rest days.

Injuries

My most serious running injury was plantar fasciitis. I was out for a month resting and stretching. I've also had some muscle pulls and strains. By far my most serious setback was a brain hemorrhage (also known as a hemorrhagic stroke) in 2002. How it happened is that I fell for no reason while I was on a training run. I got up and fell again. I was alone, but managed to walk three miles home. While walking I had double vision and some loss of peripheral vision and depth perception—all warning signs of a brain hemorrhage. I called Wayne and he got me to the hospital; I was unconscious on the way with little chance to survive.

I was in intensive care for a month. The doctors were all baffled as to how someone as fit as I was could have a stroke. They felt that my good conditioning helped me survive. But I lost peripheral vision and with it my ability to read, bike, and drive a car. I received conflicting advice from four doctors as to whether I should run again, but Wayne never doubted that I would. I was out walking and running after I had been home for a month. At first on runs I worried that I would have another stroke. Now I don't think about it.

Diet

I consider myself diet-conscious and eat fish and chicken, fruit, vegetables, grains, sweets in moderation, very little red meat, and drink black coffee during the day. I take vitamins daily. Before a race I like to eat a protein bar, for example a PowerBar®, and after a race I drink Gatorade® or chocolate milk. I also enjoy a massage after a hard workout.

Benefits

The benefits of running are much greater than I ever imagined. Running has helped keep me happy and healthy and provided a wonderful sense of achievement. I prefer to train alone. It's "my time" for achieving mental clarity and for reflection. Racing is something I like to do with my husband and family, helping to strengthen those bonds. I've met some terrific people in the running community and been able to travel all over the world. I really enjoy travel.

I'd advise anyone contemplating starting to run to consult your physician, start slow, and don't give up. You'll improve; nothing is impossible.

Current Goals

My current goal is to stay healthy so I can be consistent and maintain my pace. I don't want to lose speed too fast as I age, but at 80 I'm cutting my racing back to once a week and reducing my training.

In the Future

I want to continue to run and race and as long as I can. If I can't run, I'll walk and participate at races by volunteering.

SISTER MADONNA BUDER
June 12, 2011

Spokane, Washington

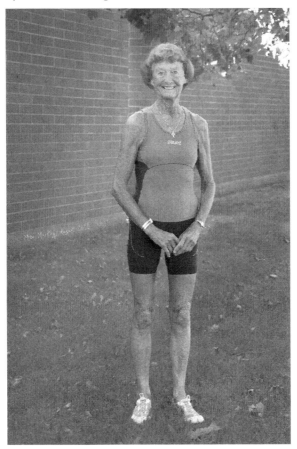

Courtesy of Mike MacKay

Age: 80

Started running: Age 48

Current training per week and long run: Varies with the season, race goal, and what else is happening in my life

Best race: Boston Marathon at age 52, 3:38; likely the oldest woman

I was given the Runner's World *2007 Heroes Award for my performance in the 2006 Hawaiian Ironman when I finished in awful weather at the age of 76. After the ceremony, another awardee—the race director of the Boston Marathon—said, "Sister, anytime you'd like to do the Boston Marathon, you're in." In 2011 I was the only woman over 80 to finish officially. (Although unconfirmed, Madonna is likely the only woman over 80 to ever finish the Boston Marathon.)*

Early Years and Family

I was born on July 24, 1930 in St. Louis, Missouri, and grew up there. I was born during a heat wave, which perhaps accounts for my ability to withstand high temperatures, and my love of the sun.

My grandfather was one of the founders of the St. Louis Opera Company, and built the landmark Buder Building near the waterfront. My father, a lawyer, went to his office in the Buder Building until he was 83. He was a champion oarsman in his younger days and played handball until he was 70. My mother was a budding actress destined for Broadway. They were opposites—a conscientious German Unitarian and an artistic, spiritual French Catholic.

As a child I was always outdoors engaging in adventurous activities like skiing, sledding, tennis, roller skating, ice skating, and mountain climbing—the oldest and only girl with three younger brothers. I became an accomplished equestrian and competed successfully in local horse shows. I enjoyed many sports that involved running, including field hockey, baseball, basketball, high jump, tennis, soccer, and the usual neighborhood games. I was on some winning teams and acquired my share of ribbons. Running as a competitive sport was not available at that time for women.

I began to receive formal instruction in the Catholic faith when I was 10 years old. At 18 I enrolled in Maryville College, then transferred to Washington University for my last two college years. After a long emotional struggle I broke a wonderful relationship with a young Irishman, choosing to join a semi-cloistered order, the Sisters of the Good Shepherd. I took my final vows at the age of 26 and was sent to convents in seven different cities counseling troubled teenage girls, eventually settling in Spokane, Washington.

Getting Started

In 1978, at the age of 48, I was introduced to running during a workshop on spirituality at Rockaway on the Oregon coast. The priest giving the workshop started talking about the benefits of running. He believed it was a joyful release, a way to harmonize the mind, body, and soul, saying how running could diminish depression, diabetes, addictions, and stress while increasing concentration. I told him that nothing could be that good. Yet, later that evening—it was April Fool's day—I put on some donated running shorts and a pair of secondhand tennis shoes and began running in the dark on the beach. It felt good. The priest spotted me as I returned, and asked me how far I had gone and how long it had taken me. I responded that I had run about a half a mile in five minutes. He seemed impressed and told me to keep it up. So I ran for the next two days during the workshop, and lingered several days longer, making a private retreat that included running on the beach.

When I returned from the beach I kept on running. Five weeks later I tried my first race, the Bloomsday Run, 8.2 miles in Spokane. When I started training, I had no idea what training was, and was still wearing my secondhand tennis shoes with thin soles, running about seven miles a day in them. After three weeks my calves were so tight I couldn't make an indentation in them. My knees were enlarged. Exhausted, I broke down and cried, then asked the Lord for strength. A benefactor of the convent came forward to buy me a proper pair of running shoes—which, because my proper size was not available, gave me blisters.

Race day was bright and clear, and the camaraderie at the back of the pack made the event feel festive. Nearly all the runners were younger than me. My goal had been to just get through the race, but by the time I finished I realized that I couldn't let go of running. I decided to run one race a month.

Once I began running and competing, I rediscovered my adventurous spirit. I went mountain and glacier climbing with my brothers. Soon after I started to run, I decided I wanted to run a marathon. Not just any marathon: the Boston Marathon. So I began training really hard, increasing my distance little by little in order to qualify. In 1982 the qualifying time for women over 40 was three hours and thirty minutes. I was already 52! To make the effort worthwhile I decided to raise money for MS. My qualifying race was the Coeur d'Alene Marathon in Idaho. I crossed the finish line with just 48 seconds to spare; at 52 I was probably one of the oldest women to qualify at that time.

On the day of the Boston Marathon, I had only a glass of milk, a banana, and granola for breakfast at 6:30 a.m.; by the time the Marathon started at noon, I was already hungry. And, I didn't take water during the race at the aid stations because I didn't want to lose time. All went well until the last four miles, when I wanted to break stride. My legs began to feel like lead, but I finished with a time of 3:38 and had raised $4,000 in pledges for MS!

Although inspired by the frontrunners at the time, I really had had no role models other than the saints and the Mother of God. I was certainly aware of Helen Klein, with whom I did an infomercial once for the HealthRider® exercise machine, and Sister Marion Irvine, who was six months older than me. We both ran the Oakland Marathon in the same year, but I never saw her tail.

By now I had discovered that I was both competitive and quite good. However, when I was peaking in my 10th year of running, I learned that there is such a thing as an addicted runner. After running high mileage (60 to 70 miles a week) with its constant pounding, I discovered what burnout was. I kept a log of my races, so I know that there were years when I was running about 20 races in one season. I had to be careful not to push myself too hard. On the other hand, not striving left no room for improvement. This was a delicate balance.

A triathlon seemed like the next natural step. The triple sports involved in the triathlon saved me from the compulsiveness that sometimes overtakes runners. Even though my running times slowed, I maintained my overall conditioning. Although I learned to dress like a triathlete to not stand out, some consider my behavior inappropriate for a Catholic nun. While Vatican II in 1962 had eased restrictions on what nuns could wear, my order continued to be very traditional. I found peace in the realization that if God gives you a talent, he expects you to use it. In the words of Christ, "You have not chosen me, but I have chosen you" (John 15:16). To me that meant that I have not chosen running and triathlons; they have chosen me. Although most races are on weekends, I have not missed Sunday Mass except when captive in an airplane crossing over the international date line.

I read a book called *Sudden Spring* by Lillanna Kopp, a former Sisters of the Holy Names nun. She described a type of sisterhood, called the Sisters for Christian Community, in which the nuns who live and work in a community make decisions by consensus. In 1986 I requested and then received, after a few years, permission to transfer there. As a nun in this community, I have the freedom to choose my own ministry and lifestyle. I now live on my own in Spokane, counseling persons in jail and doing other volunteer work.

After several years of disappointing setbacks while training for the Hawaiian Ironman, I was able to make it to Kona in 1985. As it happened, a hurricane had passed by the night before, leaving a strong ocean current with two-to-four-foot swells, causing me to miss the cutoff coming out of the water by four minutes. The next year (1986) I finished Kona with a time of 14:31:58—an age-group record for women 55 to 59. In 1987 at eight miles on the run, I realized I had fractured the metatarsal in my left foot due to a bad choice of shoes—and still finished. In 1988 I broke two toes the night before the race and finished with my slowest time to that date, 16:18:20.

By 1992 I was 62 and competing regularly in tris at the Ironman distance. I aimed for a time of under 13 hours but was thrilled with finish times of 13:16:34 for the Canadian Ironman and 13:19:01 for the Hawaiian Ironman in Kona. Not only were these times my personal bests, but I set a 13-year record for women 60 to 64. A typical spring circuit would be the Mount Rainier duathlon in western Washington in mid-April; the St. Anthony's Triathlon in St. Petersburg, Florida, at the end of April; Beat the Beast Half Ironman in St. Croix, Virgin Islands a week later, the Gulf Coast Half Ironman in Panama City, Florida, the following week; then an Olympic-distance triathlon in Memphis in May; followed by the St. Louis Senior Olympics and—finally—a duathlon in Sylvania, Ohio.

In 1995 I moved into a new age group: 65 to 69. I won this age group in order to open it for women in the Hawaiian Ironman. In 2005, I established a 75–79 age-group record in the Canadian Ironman (16:46:21) and did the same at Kona in 15:54:15. I was happy with that even though my 60–64 and 65–69 records were broken at Kona that same year.

In 2006 I won the Cannondale Determination Award (and a new Cannondale bike) at Kona for finishing in awful weather conditions at age 76. I was fine out of the water, then biked in torrential rains. My stomach was upset when I started the run and the rains continued, creating at one point a river that I didn't think I could wade across. Crowds went wild cheering me in at the finish. I made it with just 57 seconds to spare.

I was also given the *Runner's World* 2007 Heroes Award for my performance in the 2006 Hawaiian Ironman. After the ceremony, another awardee—Dave McGillivray, race director of the Boston Marathon—came to me and said, "Sister, anytime you'd like to do the Boston Marathon, you're in." I thanked him but told him that I only did marathons if they were connected to the Ironman Distance triathlons, and lately I was mostly walking, not running. Due to stomach issues, I still had not found the right nourishment for long distances.

In spite of what I told Mr. McGillivray, though, in November of 2007 I decided to run the 2008 Boston Marathon. Our winter that year in Spokane was one of the most severe and prolonged ever. By March, with the race six weeks away, I had managed to work in just three 10-mile runs when I encountered another setback: a pulled groin muscle in a bike accident. Now I couldn't run at all, just shuffle painfully. Within two weeks of the marathon I was able to fit in one five-mile run and two half marathon training runs. Hence, I toed the start line in Hopkinton with a mere total of 61 miles of training. Hardly recommended! I was amazed and overjoyed to finish in 4:42:41. I was the oldest woman to finish and third in the 70-plus women's age group!

In 2011 I was the first (and only) woman over 80 to finish the Boston Marathon. I was nearly an hour under the cutoff of six hours. Again, I had little time to train. I did nowhere near the training I needed. Fortunately, there is something magical about the Boston course. Once you start, it just pulls you forward.

I've kept records of my triathlon times but didn't start it soon enough. However, I know that I have competed in over 350 triathlons—including 45 Ironman races—as of June 2011. I have also competed regularly in road races, but far fewer since I have been doing triathlons. By now I am not only the oldest woman, but sometimes the oldest participant in these triathlons. No doubt I am slowing down. Now I can complete Ironmans under the 17-hour cutoff by only the slimmest of margins. I'll have a good swim and bike ride, but my stomach won't cooperate on the run. At one time I held four age-group records simultaneously in the Canadian Ironman.

Training Schedule

I am my own trainer using three principles: (1) I don't waste time training for training's sake; (2) I incorporate training into my daily life using my bike or running errands whenever practical; (3) I try to make it joyful with prayer and creative imagery. I've always undertrained rather than overtrained. I swim at least a mile three days a week when not interrupted by travel. I run to Mass daily. If I have time, I do floor exercises (yoga postures and stretching) before running. I avoid indoor training as much as possible because I want the joy of being outside. When I compete in one triathlon after another during the season, I figure each one is training for the next.

Injuries

Most of my injuries have been the result of bicycle accidents while training, just once during competition. I always try to ride my bike defensively. Nevertheless, on a visit to St. Louis in 1983 I had a horrific bicycle accident, flipping over the handlebars and crashing into the curb. I ended up with a compound fractured right elbow, which required screws to hold together. About a month later I ran the invitational Diet Pepsi Championship 10K in New York with a cast on my arm and sign on my back saying: INJURED RUNNER, NO PASSING ON THE RIGHT. Not long after that, when I was hoping to go to the Hawaiian Ironman, I broke my hip in another biking accident in rush-hour traffic.

Finding Time

Finding time to train has become a major problem for me. The Spokane winter weather is brutal, with snow often covering the roads. And I've been spending a lot of time giving talks and at book signings.

Current Goals

Last year I wanted to set an 80-plus female age record in both the Canadian and Hawaiian Ironmans, but I couldn't finish the Canadian Ironman because an ill-fitting wet suit interfered with my swim, and I couldn't finish a tri in Arizona because the water was unusually cold and choppy. So, I couldn't go to Hawaii because these two tris were to be my qualifier events. My goal this year is to finish both the Canadian and Hawaiian races and set the 80-plus age-group records.

Benefits

When I started I learned so much, not only about running, but about myself. Running was a new prayer form for me. At first, part of the joy in running was the being outdoors close to nature. Even now my problems shrink when I'm surrounded by God's creation. On longer runs I recite the rosary. Running not only helped me solve problems, it reduced anxiety surrounding them. It helped to free my spirit and took away brooding darkness at a time when there was a lot of turmoil in my life.

In the Future

I can't explain the desire to keep going. When I turned 60, I thought about giving it up. Then 70. Now that I'm 80, I no longer think about quitting. When people ask me how I do it I have a very simple answer: "I don't know."

If I achieve my goal of opening up 80-years-plus age groups in the Hawaiian and Canadian Ironmans, I plan to take a vacation from Ironman distances and concentrate on shorter distances. It is necessary to establish a goal to keep going. At my age, running is the hardest of the three sports. Swimming is one thing you can do forever.

Editor's Note: For additional information about Sister Madonna's life and accomplishments, see her autobiography: *The Grace to Race (with Karin Evans, Simon and Schuster, 2010).*

BETTY LUNDQUIST
Spring Hill, Florida

April 9, 2011

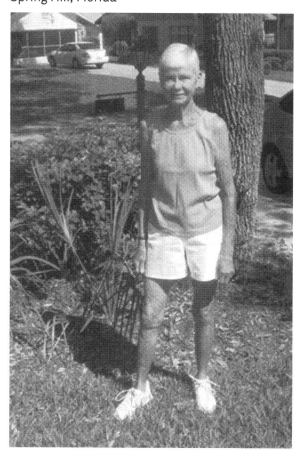

Age: 82
Started running: Age 61
Current training per week: Plays tennis up to four hours per day
Best race: A 5K under 30 minutes

My daughter thought I could run. So for my next birthday (my 61st), my daughter and son-in-law gave me tights and running shoes. This was February; it's cold in February in New Jersey. They drove me to the boardwalk, put me out, and told me to run a two-mile stretch. They didn't run with me! They just drove along, encouraging me. I had to run to stay warm

Early Years and Family

I was born in Cookeville, Tennessee, and grew up in Detroit. In terms of my ethnicity, I tell people I'm pretty much a mutt. When I was four months old, my parents moved to Detroit where my father was looking for work—this was, of course, the depression of the 1930s. He eventually found work in a roller bearing plant, in time becoming a journeyman tool-and-die maker.

I was active in sports in grade school; everyone was in those days. In high school I went out for the tennis team and made it. So few people played tennis that, if you went out, you were sure to make the team. I also went out for baseball but sprained my ankle right away and had to quit. I attended Michigan State College (now University) where I only participated in diving and fencing as part of the required gym classes. If track was available, I wasn't aware of it. I loved to swim. If I was around water I had to get in it.

I met my husband at Michigan State. He graduated with a degree in electrical engineering; my degree was in medical technology. Right after we were married, we moved to New Jersey for his job. He was from Elizabeth, New Jersey, so for him it was like going home. We had two daughters. The youngest, who lives in Denver, has a daughter now 12 years old. I worked for the local YMCA for 30 years, part-time when my girls were in school and full-time later, retiring as business manager.

Getting Started

My husband jogged for a while but never raced. I tried jogging with him to keep my weight down. I wasn't heavy and wanted to keep it that way. I couldn't keep up with him, and it became clear that he didn't want to be bothered. So I gave that up. After my husband died in 1989, I was looking around for something to do. I joined a local tennis club, took lessons, and then started playing regularly.

My oldest daughter (now 56) and her husband run, and introduced me to running. How it happened is that I was with her and my son-in-law at a race that included a one-mile fun run for children. His children were doing the fun run. As we were standing around waiting for it to start, I wondered, "How hard could it be to run a mile?" So I got into the race without the proper clothes or shoes. It was embarrassing. I was dead last. The ambulance was right behind me with somebody asking, "Are you all right, lady?" I finished, though. That experience made my daughter think that I could run.

So for my next birthday (my 61st), my daughter and son-in-law gave me tights and running shoes. This was February; it's cold in February in New Jersey.

They drove me to the boardwalk, put me out, and told me to run a two-mile stretch. They didn't run with me! They just drove along, encouraging me. I had to run to stay warm.

Progression

After my two-mile boardwalk run, I started running one mile to and from a park in my neighborhood after work. That wasn't hard, so I started running around the park too. The distance was just under 5K. I knew I could run two more blocks to make it a 5K, so I started doing that. In the spring, I decided to run the Cherry Blossom 5K in Newark, New Jersey. I was a little concerned because the race was in the morning and I had always run after work. My goal was just to finish—I hadn't thought about awards. But the awards made racing more fun because I often placed in my age group. There were so few women my age running that, in races with awards three deep, frequently fewer than three women showed up. I won a lot of medals. My daughter has hundreds.

My daughter, at 57, and my son-in-law, who is now 61, went to races almost every weekend. I started going with them or meeting them when there were races near their New Jersey shore home. My son-in-law was always telling me that, if I wanted to run faster, I had to train faster and more often. I told him, "You are giving me a good incentive to live. I want to see how you are doing at my age." The social part of running was important for my daughter and son-in-law. For me, it was being with them. Maybe because I'm an only child, I think of myself pretty much as a loner.

I never joined any running groups or read books or magazines about running. I did keep a log of my runs, and my son-in-law to whom I owe a lot for keeping me going, computerized it. I had gotten up to 2,000 miles one year, and my training runs were up to six miles. I raced 5Ks, 10Ks, 15Ks, and a few half marathons. I ran most of the races, no matter the distance, at a 10-minute-mile pace. I ran the Long Beach Island (LBI) 18-mile race once. Although I didn't realize it at the time, my kids were training me for a marathon! They made a mistake. I ran a half marathon one weekend and the LBI race the following weekend. When I got to the end of the 18 miles, I thought that there was no way I could go another eight miles. I shouldn't have done the two races so close together. I never really wanted to run a marathon, although I was intrigued at one point with the idea of going back home to Detroit for one.

All this time I was in a tennis club and played on Saturdays and Sundays. I met a man at the club when I was 66 who swept me off my feet. He wanted to marry, but my kids were concerned, feeling I should wait to be sure. He had bought a house near where I now live in Florida, so I retired and came down here to be with him. The relationship subsequently ended, but I liked living here so much that I bought my own place and stayed.

This community has a tennis club, three golf courses, and good places to run. There are two main roads: a 2.4-mile circle and a horseshoe loop of 3.6 miles encircling all the homes. I would sometimes run both. After I moved here, I ran competitively for a while. My daughter, son-in-law, and I did a few *St. Petersburg Times* Turkey Trots. I ran the 5K and they ran the 5K and the 10K. Afterwards we'd go for breakfast and hang out on the beach for a while. Some years ago, the three of us and two men from this community went together to a 10K race. We were all in different age groups. It was a killer of a race because there were a lot of hills, not typical of Florida. We all won our age groups; me, of course, because I was the only one in it. It was fun for all of us.

My last race was the Gasparilla Distance Classic in 2002. I have a cup for being in the top 10 in my age group. I'm pretty sure there weren't 10 women in my age group. When I reached the point where I couldn't do that 2.4-mile circle in at least 12-minute miles, I couldn't really call what I was doing running and gave it up.

Now I play tennis regularly and have played in tournaments. I have a number of trophies from winning mixed and ladies' doubles. I am one of only three women over 80 in my community still playing tennis and the only one who will play six sets in a row.

I've biked but not competitively. A friend from Detroit and I did seven bicycle trips in Europe with Elderhostel. The first was in 1992, a few years after my husband died. On those trips we typically spent five days biking anywhere from 20 to 40 miles between accommodations. There were always some jocks in the group and I enjoyed showing them they weren't the only ones...mild competition.

I recently took up the game of billiards. The community billiards room is nearby. I joined the women's league and won the first billiards tournament I was in. That was, by far, the most stressful thing I have ever done. You have a whole room of people watching your every move. It is much more stressful than running. I also enjoy playing ping-pong, and played here for a while. However, when I became the only woman who showed up, I felt uncomfortable playing with all men, so I stopped.

Injuries

Injuries were never a problem for me. Early on I got shin splints. Once I knew what they were and the treatment, they didn't last long.

Diet

My diet is bad. Apparently it is good for me, but I would not recommend it. For lunch I've eaten the same thing for over 20 years: extra-sharp cheese, crackers, and iced tea. For a while after my husband died, and before I started running, I didn't eat breakfast or lunch! I wasn't particularly hungry. (I made up for it at dinner.) Now for breakfast I have half a cup of cereal with half a banana sliced and grapefruit in the winter, cantaloupe in the summer. I drink tea, not coffee. For years I've had a double martini before dinner. That's all the alcohol I drink except, on rare occasions, wine. For dinner I have a large salad, pasta or potatoes or rice, and fish or meat. I stopped eating vegetables years ago because it is too difficult to keep good fresh vegetables on hand without shopping every couple of days. I don't like sweets. If I have a craving after dinner I eat a few handfuls of nuts.

I have taken Centrum® One-A-Day for years and now Centrum® Silver. I don't use energy drinks because they are invariably sweet. I usually rely on plain water.

Benefits

I do feel that sports give me a lift emotionally. I feel good about what I've accomplished and that I can still keep playing. There is one point that I feel strongly about people knowing. When I started running, my son-in-law said to me, "Mom, I can't promise that running will extend your life, but I promise running will extend your active life." That is *so* true.

I have plenty of energy. I enjoy yard work, although I've noticed that I can't do it for as long as I once did. I'm also getting a little leery of being on a ladder. Longevity now is the luck of the draw. My only health problem is slightly high blood pressure, which I take medication for.

Current Goal

I'm planning to drive to my daughter's house in Maine this summer, then fly to my 65th high school reunion in Michigan, visit my other daughter in Denver, fly back to Maine, and drive home to Florida.

JACKIE YOST
Treasure Island, Florida

February 10, 2011

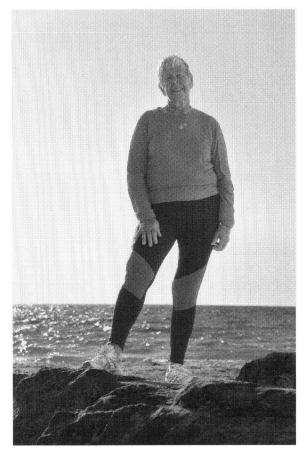

Courtesy of Mike MacKay

Age: 83
Started running: In my 40s
Current training per week: 15–20 miles including race walking and jogging
Long run: Up to 7 miles depending on training goal
Best race: Ford Ironman 70.3 World Championship at age 78

We'd do the St. Anthony's Olympic distance triathlon in St. Petersburg most years. We have been out in Tampa Bay where the swimming part takes place, when it has been rough. But when the whistle blows you just do it. It's time to go. You Show, Go, and Finish.

Early Years and Family

I was born in Thomasville, North Carolina, and grew up there. My parents were not athletic themselves but they encouraged and supported me in whatever I wanted to do. In high school we had a physical education teacher from the Women's College of the University of North Carolina (WC-UNC) who frequently invited her instructors to give talks to her classes. Hearing them, I thought, "This is what I want to do." I owe so much to my parents and to my school.

So I went to WC-NUC in Greensboro when it was ranked third in the nation for majors in women's physical education. In that era we could not specialize in one sport. It is different now. For the first two years we had 16 hours of physical education in addition to a full course load. We were taught and participated in all the sports through intramural games. If you did well in those games you were chosen to represent the college in intercollegiate games. The faculty was excellent, but had high expectations. We were expected to excel not only at sports but academically. The members of the faculty were my role models. They wanted us to go into the community and instill fitness goals in others.

In retrospect I believe it was good to try all sports. I learned what was available and was able to teach many different sports. The philosophy was to reach as many children as possible within the schools, emphasizing intramural teams. Being a graduate of the UNC-WC physical education department opened a lot of doors for me. My first job was recreation center director, Winston-Salem, North Carolina. In that position I had to teach swimming, baseball, tennis, softball, basketball, whatever. Subsequently, I was girls' athletic director and coach and kindergarten teacher at Methodist Orphanage in Raleigh, North Carolina, and from 1961–1980 taught health, science, and physical education in Virginia, Georgia, and Florida.

I have been married to my husband Larry, an accomplished runner and triathlete, for 58 years. We have three children and two grandchildren. The children, now in their 50s, and the grandchildren, who are in their 20s, are all triathletes. We are very, very proud of that fact. We have passed it on.

Getting Started

So, although sports have been a major part of my life since childhood, I did not start running until much later. Track and field was only a small part of the WC-UNC program and it was not stressed. Between raising children and starting to run, I played golf with friends and also competitively. When we moved to Florida I decided to give up golf—with some reluctance. I had started running in the 1970s and continued to run. My first race was a 5K in Clemson, South Carolina, in 1978. I won my age group! That's what motivated me to continue! I ran my best times then—with no coach, didn't know what I was doing really. I did my first five-mile race that year too. I went with a group of my golfing friends who were all much younger than me. I kept up with them, and I remember thinking, "This is fun." I've always enjoyed running; training is not hard work for me.

Progression

Larry started running a few years before I did. He would be running miles and I was just running around a track at first. We were not around other runners, didn't have a coach for advice, so I progressed by increments, running the same distance in increasingly faster times. We did not read about running until later. We've always done things together, so it was natural that we started going to road races together.

My daughter Joy and I started a little business called Energetics Unlimited when we moved to Florida in 1980. She had just graduated from the University of Florida with a recreation degree. We decided that we would offer services such as aerobics and sports training to condo dwellers. The idea was to provide exercise activities that otherwise would require the residents to go elsewhere, such as a gym, to find. We were a little ahead of the times. There were only a few takers. A year and half later all the condo associations wanted these services. Unfortunately, by that time my daughter had moved on. She needed a larger income. And Larry and I had gotten involved in property management.

Larry has run several marathons. I have raced all distances up to and including the half marathon, never a marathon. That would take too much time to prepare for and to run. I like to finish without feeling totally exhausted. We have run in all the Disney Half Marathons except the first and the last two. We've been doing the Gasparilla 15K since 1980 or 1981. We belong to the St. Pete Beach Road Runners Club and run their summer series. I don't routinely keep a log of my races. I'll look back in the published race results sometimes to see what I've done in a race the previous year. I've finished in the top five in my age group in all events.

I started doing triathlons in 1993, when I was 65. After we moved here we were asked to join the St. Pete MAD DOGS Triathlon Club. Our friends kept after us to join them and to try a triathlon. The club had a short triathlon for newbies called the Meek and the Mighty. Larry and I discussed it and decided that, since they kept asking us, we'd give it a try. So we did and we liked it. The next year we decided we didn't want to do the short one; we'd do the St. Anthony's Olympic-distance tri in St. Petersburg. And we've been doing it most years since. We have been out in Tampa Bay where the swimming part takes place, when it has been rough. But when the whistle blows you just do it. It's time to go. You Show, Go, and Finish.

MAD DOGS is a close-knit group. We enjoy the camaraderie. We watch out for each other. We look to other members for advice, and for recommendations of medical practitioners if we need them. Some of the MAD DOGS are physicians. A group of us practices swimming in the Gulf of Mexico off our Treasure Island home every Friday morning at 8 a.m. It is not as difficult as you might think. To get started you just do what you can. You go out with the group, go as far as you can, and then see where the rest of the group has gotten. Then go a little farther the next time. You increase incrementally, just like in running. We wear wet suits early and late in the season. The water gets warm very quickly. It's so refreshing. In fact, the thrill of swimming, biking, and running was so great that I looked forward to every race. Olympic and sprint distances are my specialties.

We were doing 12–15 triathlons every year, and road races, until I had my open-heart surgery. So we were doing an event almost every weekend. I win my age group if Sister Madonna Buder does not show up. Sister Madonna has been doing triathlons for many years. She is one of the oldest women to have done Kona and goes to all the major triathlons. Her combination of body build, ability, agility, and stamina make her great. She's tops in my age group in the country. If I lose to anyone, she is the one I want to lose to.

Editor's Note: Jackie's running and triathlon championships over a 30-plus-year career are too numerous to list here. She has placed first in her age group at the Disney Half Marathon, the Gasparilla distance Classic 15K, St. Anthony's Triathlon (Olympic Distance), Disney Minnie Marathon 15K, and second at the Ford Ironman 70.3 World Championship. In addition she has been consistently ranked first or second in her age group by USA Triathlon, the national triathlon governing body. She was a USAT Age-Group ALL AMERICAN in 1998–99, 2001–4, 2006, and 2009.

We still enjoy playing golf, and take summer memberships on certain golf courses. Since there are not many people here in the summer, it is like having the whole course to yourself. We walk, rather than take a cart. Walking is another favorite activity.

Injuries

There was one other female runner about my age in the area, but she dropped out about five years ago. I guess people stop running simply because their bodies break down. I've been blessed in that I've not had running injuries or even aches and pains. I broke my clavicle once when a nonparticipating man on a bike rode across the bike path in front of me during the bike part of a triathlon, and I crashed. I healed in six weeks—no big deal.

Health

I started to slow down dramatically about three years ago. I was given a stress test that the doctor had to stop after two minutes! Previously, I'd passed stress tests with flying colors. The cause was a leaking heart valve that needed to be either repaired or replaced. Fortunately, they were able to repair it during surgery, and to also fix a small hole in my heart. I started to move as soon as possible during my convalescence. I used the elliptical machine at first. I now am back to swimming and biking, but I can't run like I used to. So I've taken up race walking. This year I'll have to do the 5K rather than the 15K at Gasparilla, and that is hard emotionally.

Larry and I do everything together except that I can no longer run with him. We used to start and finish on the beach. We had done our bike rides with the MAD DOG group downtown in St. Petersburg. However, there were so many accidents, I decided that was too dangerous and, after surgery, we have been taking our bikes out to Fort De Soto Park. You can get in 56 miles there and it is safe. We go to a local gym for weightlifting. We don't go as often as we should because there is so much else to do. To find time to train, we go to bed very early and get up very early (5 a.m.). We do most of our athletic activities and property management in the morning. I have never enjoyed working out in the afternoon. Too tired. Larry and I believe that we are the oldest triathlon couple in the country.

Two afternoons a week I go out for a two-mile race walk. I practice parts of it like heels, toes, rocking. Race walking is not normal. Until it becomes normal for me I'll never be any good. I've been doing it for over two years, taking a class from a woman who teaches progressively, the way I believe in.

She teaches one skill for a week, then adds another skill the next week. The students advance from Beginners to Intermediate to Advanced classes. We're never too old to learn. My race walking instructor stresses stretching. We never end a class without stretching, and she emphasizes that we must do it on our own. It helps.

Last year we went to New Orleans to do a half Ironman relay. Our daughter Cindy did the half Ironman on her own. Larry, our daughter Joy, and I did the half Ironman as a relay. I did the 56-mile bike part. This year at St. Anthony's, for the first time, I'll do a relay. Right now my goal is to participate. I want to be part of the game. It's not for competition. I enjoy it so much I can't stop. My son Steve, his wife, and their daughter do that race as a relay too.

Training Schedule

Our weekly schedule is:

Monday: spinning or biking when the weather is good, and pool swimming
Tuesday: track for speed work
Wednesday: biking and pool swimming
Thursday: long run/race walk
Friday: open-water swim, coffee for athletes afterwards
Saturday: weights, and sometimes fit them in other days
Sunday: long run/race walk, adding a mile over Thursday

Diet

I have to be careful with my diet. I eat a lot of fruits and vegetables. I slip, which I think is normal. I eat small amounts of protein but not as much fish as I'd like. We use an energy drink called Metabolol mixed with orange juice before we go out in the morning. Sometimes we'll take a GU. We'll use Gatorade® as a supplement when we are biking and swimming.

I take fish oil and a multivitamin. I take Flexcin®, a glucosamine-based supplement. The Flexcin® creator asked to sponsor me several years ago and gave me some. I found it to be great. My joints just worked better after I started taking it. I have continued even after the sponsorship ended. Larry takes it too.

In the Future

I'm not concerned about living long, but I want to be healthy as long as I'm living. I expect to participate in races as long as I can. It is up to me to make myself improve. No one can do it for me. If it means harder work, I work harder. Race walking is definitely harder.

I do believe that the swimming and biking have helped my running. They make running easier, and I don't know if I would have been able to continue running as long as I have if I were not also biking and swimming.

Postscript

I decided in early 2012 that maybe I *am* too old to learn race walking. I wasn't improving. So I decided to go back to running; It's more natural. At first I ran three minutes, walked three minutes for a mile; then I progressed to run three minutes, walk two minutes for a mile. Next I started doing one mile of run three, walk three alternating with a mile of run three, walk two until I could go four miles. I progressed to the track where I'm running six 200-meter repeats followed by six 100s. After about six weeks I can run 5Ks! I'm so excited.

Events

Avon International Marathon: A women-only marathon first held in 1978 in Atlanta, Georgia. Drawing 186 outstanding women from nine nations, it was important in proving that women had equal rights to distance sports.

Boston Marathon: Notable for the requirement to qualify by meeting the designated time standard that corresponds with the runner's age and gender. In 2012, because of the large number of runners applying, for the first time acceptance will take place in stages, with the fastest qualifiers in relation to their qualifying time standard being accepted first until the race is full. In 2011, registration was closed before many qualifiers could register. It is also possible to run the marathon by raising money for a charity.

Broad Street Run: A 10-mile point-to-point race down a major Philadelphia, Pennsylvania thoroughfare held the first Sunday in May. First run in 1980, it is the largest 10-miler in the United States and one of the fastest races.

Escape from Alcatraz Triathlon: 1.5-mile swim through the cold waters of San Francisco Bay from Alcatraz island to shore, 18-mile bike race, and 8-mile run through rugged trails. An extreme event in its 32nd year in 2012. Entrants may qualify or be selected by lottery.

Gasparilla Distance Classic: A large 15K race held annually in Tampa, Florida at the end of February/first of March. Associated with Tampa's Gasparilla Pirate Festival.

Grand Prix: A series of races in which both individuals and teams compete, with awards given according to performances in all races.

Ironman World Championship Triathlon in Kona, Hawaii: To compete, athletes must win a spot through the lottery, or earn one at one of the qualifying events held around the world. Tens of thousands compete for one of 1,800 spots.

Meek and the Mighty Triathlon: 100-yard swim, 3.6-miles cycle ride, half-mile run (ages 7 to 10); 200-yard swim, 5.4-mile cycle ride, and 1-mile run (ages 11 and over). Held in conjunction with St. Anthony's Triathlon.

Philadelphia Distance Run (now Philadelphia Rock 'n' Roll Half Marathon): A large half marathon held in Philadelphia in mid-September.

St. Anthony's Triathlon: A major Olympic-distance triathlon held in downtown St. Petersburg, Florida, at the end of April.

Susan G. Komen Race for the Cure: A race/walk event held in numerous (146 in 2011) cities and international locations throughout the year to fund primarily breast-cancer research, education, advocacy, and services. Since 1983 there have been well over one million participants and nearly two billion dollars have been raised.

Trevira Twosome: A 10-mile road race held in New York's Central Park, in which men and women are paired, with times combined.

Half-Ironman Triathlon: 1.2-mile swim, 56-mile cycle ride, 13.1-mile run.

Ironman Triathlon: 2.4-mile swim, 112-mile cycle ride, 26.2-mile run.

Olympic-Distance Triathlon: 1500-meter swim, 40-kilometer cycle ride, 10-kilometer run.

Sprint-Distance Triathlon: 750-meter swim, a 20-kilometer cycle ride, 5-kilometer run.

Elite Women Runners

Madonna Buder and Harriet Anderson: Both women have won their age group in Kona through their 60s and 70s; both have finished despite injuries or illness; and both have been the oldest female finisher in the race.

Marion Irvine: A nun, now over 80, who ran in the Olympic Trials at the age of 54.

Helen Klein:: Well-known in the running community for running ultra-marathons into her 70s. Over 80 and still running.

Ingrid Kristiansen: A Norwegian born in 1956 who was one of the best female long-distance runners of her time.

Joan Benoit Samuelson: Female winner of the 1984 Olympic Marathon, the first year the event was open to women. Arguably the best-known and most inspirational female distance runner in the United States, she continues to compete at a very high level, setting age-group records in her 50s.

Kathrine Switzer: Born in 1947, a pioneer in women's distance running in the United States. Best known for being the first woman to compete officially in the Boston Marathon (she used her initials on the entry form in 1967), where the race director tried to forcibly remove her from the course. She won the New York City Marathon in 1974, and continues a successful career promoting and supporting women's running.

Grete Waitz: Born in Norway in 1953, Grete won nine New York City Marathons between 1978 and 1988, more than any other runner. She was second to Joan Benoit in the 1984 Olympics. Sadly, she died of cancer in 2011.

Priscilla Welch: A record-setting British masters runner who took up running later in life. In 1987 she won the New York City Marathon in 2:30:17 at nearly 43 years of age. The following spring she set the masters record at Boston in 2:30:48, a mark that stood until 2002.

Injuries and Anatomy

Anterior Cruciate Ligament (ACL): One of four major knee ligaments. The ACL is critical to knee stability.

Iliotibial Band (ITB): A superficial thickening of tissue on the outside of the thigh, extending from the outside of the pelvis, over the hip and knee, and inserting just below the knee.

Piriformis Syndrome (also known as **Sciatica**)**:** A condition in which the piriformis, a narrow muscle located in the buttocks, irritates the sciatic nerve, causing pain in the buttocks and referring pain and numbness along the course of the sciatic nerve to the foot.

Plantar Fasciitis: Irritation and swelling of the thick tissue on the bottom of the foot. The most common complaint is pain on the bottom of the heel.

Shin Splints: Pain in your shin bones (the larger of the two bones below your knee). A common running injury caused by swollen muscles, stress fractures, or flat feet.

Energy Drinks, Foods and Supplements

Clif Shot Bloks®: Chewable cubes with both carbohydrates and electrolytes.

Cytomax®: An energy drink made of complex carbohydrates and sugars.

Endurolytes® (a Hammer Nutrition® product): Electrolyte supplement. Powder or capsules.

Flexcin®: A joint supplement designed to decrease inflammation and increase mobility and flexibility.

Glucosamine: A supplement used to treat osteoarthritis. Supports the structure and function of joints.

Gookinaid: See Vitalyte.

GU: A concentrated energy gel that comes in small packets and is easy to digest.

Hammer Nutrition®: A company that produces a wide variety of energy products for endurance athletes.

HEED® Sports Drink (a Hammer Nutrition® product): A sports drink with both carbohydrates and electrolytes.

Hyaluronic Acid: A substance found in the tissue space and the synovial fluid of joints that acts as a lubricating and protective agent. Taken either orally or by injection.

Metabolol: A meal replacement drink designed to improve recovery and boost energy.

Perpetuem® (a Hammer Nutrition® product): Endurance drink containing complex carbohydrates, GMO-free soy protein, healthy fats, and auxiliary nutrients such as sodium phosphate. Used by ultra-runners and others who need fuel for long periods of time.

Powerade®: Widely available sports drink for electrolyte replacement.

Vitalyte® (formerly Gookinaid): An electrolyte replacement drink.

Training/Therapy Techniques

Active Release Technique: Commonly used to treat conditions related to adhesions or scar tissue in overused muscles. Using hand pressure, the practitioner works to remove or break up the fibrous adhesions, with the stretching motions generally in the direction of venous and lymphatic flow.

Bosu: An intense total workout with an emphasis on balance.

Chi Running: No simple definition. See *Chi Running: A Revolutionary Approach to Effortless, Injury-Free Running* (Danny Dreyer and Katherine Dreyer, Fireside, May 5, 2009).

Dead Lift: Squatting down and lifting a weight off the floor with the hand until standing up straight again.

Furman Institute of Running and Scientific Training (FIRST) Program: Very simply, running specific workouts (one speed workout, one tempo run, one long run) three days a week and cross-training two or three other days.

Gallowaying: A run/walk training program, often used by beginning runners. Popularized in the United States by Jeff Galloway, a former elite runner.

Girls on the Run: A nonprofit program that helps preteen girls develop self-respect and healthy lifestyles through running.

Graston Technique: Utilizes specially designed stainless-steel instruments to specifically detect and effectively treat areas exhibiting soft-tissue fibrosis or chronic inflammation. Breaks down scar tissue.

Max VO2: The maximum capacity of an individual's body to transport and use oxygen during highest-intensity exercise; reflects the physical fitness of the individual.

Spinning: A form of indoor cycling done classroom-style with an instructor and music.

Tapering: The practice of reducing exercise in the days or weeks just before an important competition.

Team In Training (TNT): This Leukemia and Lymphoma Society program has trained nearly half a million runners, walkers, triathletes, cyclists, and hikers who have raised money for cancer research.

Shoes

Power Bounce™ Inserts: Placed in the midsole beneath the heel to create a shoe that changes in response to the speed of the runner. They improve cushioning at slow speeds, and increase the elasticity and energy return at faster speeds.

Superfeet® Orthotics: Insoles that provide support and stability.

Vibram FiveFingers®: A minimalist running shoe with a (relatively) thin rubber sole, flexible fabric top, and spaces for each toe. Integral to the barefoot running movement.

Miscellaneous

Age-graded Scores: A method for comparing race times of runners of all ages and sexes, as well as to the standard for an age and gender. A runner's age-graded score is the ratio of the approximate world-record time for the age and gender divided by his or her actual time.

Athlinks: A social networking web site that consolidates results of road races and other endurance sports.

Amby Burfoot: Editor at *Runner's World* well-known for his books and articles about running. Winner of the 1968 Boston Marathon.

DNF: An abbreviation for **D**id **N**ot **F**inish. This happens when a runner starts a race and then drops out.

Fort de Soto Park: A large and beautiful park in Pinellas County, Florida with many miles of trails.

Johnny King-Marino: A chiropractor in the Philadelphia, Pennsylvania area noted for his treatment of endurance athletes. Also a marathoner and accomplished triathlete.

The Loop: An 8.4-mile run from the Philadelphia (Pennsylvania) Art Museum, out one way along the Schuylkill River, crossing the bridge in the East Falls section of the city, and back the other side.

MAD DOGS Triathlon Club: An organization in St. Petersburg, Florida dedicated to promoting the sport of triathlon. The club is comprised of fun-loving triathletes who train, race, and howl together with members of all levels of experience and expertise. In its seventeenth year (2011) the club had 3,000-plus members throughout the country and the world.

Runner's World: A monthly publication that is read widely by runners.

Sag Wagon: A vehicle, often an ambulance or police car, following the last person in a race. The purpose is to help any runners in trouble and to signal at the finish line that the race is over.

Made in the USA
Lexington, KY
08 October 2012